The Natural Remedy Revolution
A Guide to Cancer Treatments Your Doctor May Not Share

By Karl Swarthout

ISBN: 978-1-300-92336-7

Legal Disclaimer

The information provided in this book, *The Natural Remedy Revolution A Guide to Cancer Treatments Your Doctor May Not Share* is for educational and informational purposes only. It is not intended to replace professional medical advice, diagnosis, or treatment. Always seek the guidance of your physician or other qualified healthcare provider with any questions you may have regarding a medical condition or treatment.

The author and publisher are not licensed healthcare professionals, and the information presented in this book should not be used as a substitute for medical advice from a licensed professional. The methods and strategies discussed in this book are based on research, personal experience, and expert opinion. However, individual responses to these treatments may vary, and there is no guarantee of specific outcomes. Furthermore, this book does not claim to prevent, diagnose, treat, or cure cancer. Alternative treatments, while they may offer benefits, are not a replacement for conventional medical care. Readers are encouraged to consult their healthcare providers before starting any new treatment, including the use of supplements, herbal remedies, dietary changes, or mind-body practices.

The author and publisher disclaim any liability for the decisions made by readers based on the information provided in this book. Use of the information is at the reader's own risk.

Author's Note

In a world where conventional treatments for serious illnesses like cancer often bring as many questions as answers, I felt a need to explore alternative approaches that might offer support and relief. Over the years, I've witnessed both the power and limitations of modern medicine, and I became increasingly curious about what natural, holistic remedies could do in complementing traditional treatments or even standing on their own.

The Natural Remedy Revolution is the result of extensive research, personal experiences, and a deep commitment to sharing knowledge that might benefit those seeking more control over their health. My goal in writing this book was not to dissuade anyone from seeking medical help, but rather to empower readers with options—scientifically backed natural treatments and lifestyle practices that support healing from the inside out. Here, you'll find insights on everything from nutrition and herbal remedies to mind-body practices and immune support, each one carefully examined and thoughtfully presented.

I hope that this book becomes a source of hope, knowledge, and practical guidance for you or your loved ones. May it inspire you to take small steps that could lead to powerful changes, allowing your body to work as an ally in your journey toward wellness.

Thank you for joining me in this revolution toward natural healing.

Introduction

- In an age where health challenges loom large and medical treatments evolve, a timeless truth remains prevention is often the best cure. This book aims to empower readers with comprehensive guidance on cancer prevention through the dual lenses of nutrition and holistic medicine. Beyond prevention, it offers natural remedies for those already navigating a cancer diagnosis.

- At its core, this book introduces a holistic approach to health—one that transcends isolated treatments to embrace the profound interconnectedness of diet, lifestyle choices, and natural therapies. By exploring evidence-based practices and the wisdom of holistic medicine, readers will discover practical steps to fortify their body's defenses and foster a resilient state of well-being.

- Join us on a journey where knowledge meets empowerment, where proactive choices pave the way for a healthier tomorrow. Together, let's navigate the intricate pathways of health, armed with insights that bridge the gap between traditional wisdom and contemporary science. This book is your companion in the pursuit of a life enriched by vitality and informed by the healing power of nature.

The politics of cancer treatment and the influence of Big Pharma are complex and deeply intertwined topics. Here is an overview of the key issues often discussed in this context:

Influence of Big Pharma:

Drug Pricing and Accessibility: One of the most contentious issues is the high cost of cancer drugs, which can be prohibitively expensive. Critics argue that pharmaceutical companies prioritize profits over patient access, leading to life-saving treatments being unaffordable for many.

Research Funding: Big Pharma plays a significant role in funding cancer research, which can influence the direction of research. There's concern that pharmaceutical companies may prioritize developing drugs that are more profitable rather than those that are necessarily more effective or accessible.

Clinical Trials and Regulation: Pharmaceutical companies often fund clinical trials, which can lead to potential conflicts of interest. There are concerns that negative trial results may be suppressed or that trials are designed in ways that favor positive outcomes for the drugs being tested.

Treatment Approaches:

Focus on Pharmaceuticals Over Holistic Approaches: The dominant cancer treatment model focuses on surgery, radiation, and chemotherapy. Some argue that there's not enough emphasis on prevention, lifestyle changes, or alternative therapies, partly due to the pharmaceutical industry's influence.

Patenting and Generic Drugs: Big Pharma companies often patent new drugs, which can delay the introduction of cheaper, generic versions. This patent system is a double-edged sword—it incentivizes innovation but also keeps drug prices high.

Government and Regulatory Bodies:

Regulatory Capture: There's concern about regulatory capture, where agencies like the FDA may be influenced by the industries they are supposed to regulate. This can lead to the approval of drugs that may not be the most effective or safe, but that benefit the pharmaceutical companies financially.

Lobbying and Political Influence: Big Pharma is one of the most powerful lobbying forces in many countries, particularly in the United States. Their lobbying efforts can shape healthcare policies, influence drug approval processes, and impact decisions about what treatments are covered by insurance.

Ethical Considerations:

Patient Rights and Informed Consent: The relationship between Big Pharma and the medical community raises ethical concerns about patient rights. Patients need access to unbiased information to make informed decisions about their treatment options.

Conflicts of Interest: The financial ties between pharmaceutical companies, doctors, and researchers can lead to conflicts of interest, where the best interests of the patient may not always be the primary concern.

Public Perception and Mistrust:

Mistrust in the Medical System: The influence of Big Pharma on cancer treatment contributes to public mistrust of the medical system This mistrust can lead to hesitancy in seeking conventional treatments and an increase in interest in alternative therapies.

The Role of Media: Media coverage of Big Pharma's role in cancer treatment can be polarized, with some outlets highlighting breakthroughs and others focusing on the negative aspects, such as profiteering and corruption.

The Future of Cancer Treatment:

> *Personalized Medicine:* Advances in genomics and personalized medicine offer hope for more targeted and effective cancer treatments. However, these treatments are often expensive, and there's concern that they may not be accessible to all patients.

> *Public and Private Partnerships:* There is a growing push for more collaboration between public research institutions and private companies to develop new treatments. These partnerships can be beneficial but also raise questions about who benefits most—patients or companies.

Books & Resources:

For a deeper dive into these topics, you might consider reading books such as:

"Cancer: **The Emperor of All Maladies" by Siddhartha Mukherjee**: Offers a comprehensive history of cancer treatment, including the role of pharmaceutical companies.

"*Bad Pharma:* **How Medicine is Broken, and How We Can Fix It" by Ben Goldacre**: Critically examines the pharmaceutical industry and its impact on healthcare.

These resources can provide additional context and insights into the complex relationship between cancer treatment and Big Pharma.

History of Cancer

The history of cancer is marked by a gradual evolution from mystical explanations to a scientific understanding based on cellular pathology. Early treatments were often rudimentary and invasive, but significant advancements in surgery, radiation, and chemotherapy have transformed cancer treatment. Modern approaches focus on precision medicine, targeted therapies, and harnessing the immune system, offering hope for more effective and less invasive treatments in the future.

Ancient Egypt (3000 BC):

The earliest description of cancer was found in the Edwin Smith Papyrus, an ancient Egyptian medical text. It described breast tumors that were treated by cauterization.

Ancient Greece (460-370 BC):

Hippocrates, known as the "Father of Medicine," used the terms "carcinos" and "carcinoma" to describe tumors, derived from the Greek word for crab, reflecting the appearance of the tumors.

Roman Contributions:

Aulus Cornelius Celsus (25 BC - 50 AD): Documented the first surgical treatments for cancer. He emphasized the importance of removing the tumor completely, though many treatments were rudimentary and often harmful.
Galen (130-200 AD): Proposed the humoral theory, which suggested that an imbalance of the body's four humors (blood, phlegm, yellow bile, and black bile) caused cancer. This theory dominated medical thought for centuries.

Middle Ages to Renaissance:

Limited Progress: During the Middle Ages, medical practice was heavily influenced by religion and superstition, leading to limited advancements in cancer understanding and treatment.

Renaissance (14th-17th Centuries): The Renaissance period saw a resurgence in scientific inquiry and anatomical studies. Andreas Vesalius' anatomical studies laid the groundwork for modern pathology.

18th and 19th Centuries:

Pathological Advances: Giovanni Battista Morgagni (1682-1771) linked diseases to specific organs, moving away from humoral theory.
John Hunter (1728-1793): Suggested that some cancers might be cured by surgery if they were detected early enough.

Microscopic Studies:

Rudolf Virchow (1821-1902): Known as the "Father of Modern Pathology," he identified that cells, not humors, were the source of cancer. His work established the cellular theory of cancer.

Early 20th Century:

Radiation Therapy: Wilhelm Conrad Roentgen (1895) discovered X-rays, leading to the use of radiation in diagnosing and treating cancer.
Marie and Pierre Curie (1898) discovered radium, which was used in early radiation therapies.

Surgical Advances:

William Stewart Halsted (1852-1922) developed radical mastectomy, a surgical procedure for breast cancer that became a standard treatment for many years.

Chemotherapy:

World War II and After: The use of nitrogen mustard as a chemical weapon led to the discovery of its potential to treat cancer, marking the beginning of chemotherapy. Sidney Farber's work with aminopterin, a precursor to methotrexate, showed the potential of drugs to induce remission in leukemia patients.

Modern Era:

Targeted Therapies and Immunotherapy: Since the 1970s, development of targeted therapies that focus on specific genetic mutations in cancer cells has advanced. Immunotherapy, which uses the body's immune system to fight cancer, has shown promise in treating various cancers.

Personalized Medicine:

Advances in genomics and biotechnology have led to personalized cancer treatments tailored to the genetic profile of individual tumors.

Genomic Profiling

Genomic sequencing technologies allow researchers and clinicians to analyze the DNA of cancer cells in detail. This provides insights into the specific mutations and genetic alterations driving the growth of individual tumors.

Identification of Biomarkers: By analyzing the genetic profile of tumors, specific biomarkers can be identified. Biomarkers are genetic mutations, gene expressions, or protein levels that can indicate the likelihood of a tumor responding to a particular treatment. For example, mutations like EGFR in lung cancer or HER2/neu in breast cancer can guide treatment decisions.

Targeted Therapies: Once biomarkers are identified through genomic profiling, targeted therapies can be selected. These therapies are designed to specifically target the molecular changes that drive cancer growth while minimizing damage to normal cells. Examples include tyrosine kinase inhibitors (TKIs) for tumors with specific mutations such as BRAF inhibitors for melanoma.

Immunotherapy: Genomics has also contributed to the development of immunotherapy, which harnesses the body's immune system to fight cancer. By understanding the genetic basis of tumors, researchers can develop immunotherapies that target specific antigens or enhance immune responses against cancer cells.

Precision and Effectiveness: Personalized cancer treatment improves outcomes by matching therapies to the unique genetic makeup of each patient's tumor. This approach often leads to more effective treatment with fewer side effects compared to traditional chemotherapy, which can be less selective and more broadly toxic.

Clinical Trials and Research: Genomics has accelerated clinical trials by allowing researchers to enroll patients based on their tumor's genetic profile. This can lead to faster identification of effective treatments and expand the options available to patients through targeted therapies.

Genomics and biotechnology have empowered oncologists to move beyond a one-size-fits-all approach to cancer treatment. By tailoring therapies to the genetic profile of individual tumors, personalized medicine holds promise for improving patient outcomes and transforming the landscape of cancer care.

Mechanisms of detection

Early detection of cancer is critical because it significantly increases the chances of successful treatment and survival. Recent breakthroughs in this area focus on developing non-invasive, highly accurate methods to identify cancer at its earliest stages, often before symptoms appear.

Multi-Cancer Blood Tests

One of the most exciting developments is a new blood test that can detect multiple types of cancer from a single sample. Researchers have created tests that analyze protein markers in the blood to identify 18 different cancers with high accuracy. In trials, these tests detected 93% of stage 1 cancers in men and 84% in women, offering a promising tool for widespread cancer screening. This test could become a routine part of medical checkups, allowing for early intervention when treatment is most effective.

Liquid Biopsies

Liquid biopsy technology, which involves analyzing circulating tumor DNA (ctDNA) in the blood, is another significant advance. These tests can detect mutations or other genetic changes associated with cancer, often before a tumor is visible on imaging scans. Liquid biopsies are less invasive than traditional biopsies and can be used to monitor cancer progression or recurrence after treatment.

AI-Enhanced Imaging

Artificial intelligence (AI) is also playing a crucial role in early detection. AI algorithms can analyze imaging data, such as mammograms or CT scans, to identify suspicious areas that might be missed by human radiologists. This technology is especially beneficial in regions with limited access to specialists, improving the accuracy and speed of diagnosis.

Improved Screening for Specific Cancers

For cancers like kidney cancer, improvements in imaging technology have led to earlier and more frequent incidental detection. This means that more cases are being caught in the early stages when they are more treatable. The rise in early detection has been linked to a significant decrease in mortality rates for certain cancers, such as kidney cancer, where deaths have been decreasing by about 2% annually since 2016.

These advancements in early detection are crucial steps toward reducing cancer mortality by enabling earlier, less invasive, and more effective treatment.

Understanding Cancer Formation

What is Cancer?

Cancer is a complex group of diseases characterized by the uncontrolled growth and spread of abnormal cells. Unlike normal cells, which grow, divide, and die in an orderly fashion, cancer cells continue to grow and divide uncontrollably, often forming masses of tissue called tumors. These tumors can invade surrounding tissues and spread to other parts of the body through the bloodstream or lymphatic system, a process known as metastasis.

Cancer formation, also known as carcinogenesis, is a multistep process that can be started by a variety of factors, including:

Genetic Mutations: Mutations in certain genes, such as oncogenes (which promote cell growth) and tumor suppressor genes (which inhibit cell growth), can lead to the uncontrolled cell division seen in cancer. These mutations can be inherited or acquired due to environmental factors.

Environmental Exposures: Carcinogens, which are substances capable of causing cancer, can come from a variety of sources. Common carcinogens include tobacco smoke, radiation, certain chemicals, and asbestos.

Lifestyle Factors: Diet, physical inactivity, alcohol consumption, and obesity are lifestyle factors that can increase cancer risk. For example, a diet high in red and processed meats has been linked to colorectal cancer, while a sedentary lifestyle and obesity are associated with several types of cancer, including breast and endometrial cancer.

Infections: Certain viruses and bacteria can contribute to cancer development. For example, the human papillomavirus (HPV) is linked to cervical cancer, and Helicobacter pylori infection is associated with stomach cancer.

Immune System Dysfunction: A weakened immune system, due to conditions like HIV/AIDS or immunosuppressive medications, can increase the risk of cancers, particularly those associated with viral infections.

The Process of Cancer Formation

The process of cancer formation typically involves several stages:

Initiation: This is the first step, where a normal cell undergoes genetic changes due to exposure to a carcinogen or other factors. These changes might result in the activation of oncogenes or the inactivation of tumor suppressor genes.

Promotion: During this stage, the initiated cells are stimulated to divide and grow. Factors such as chronic inflammation or hormonal imbalances can promote this abnormal cell growth.

Progression: This stage involves further genetic changes that allow the cancer cells to grow more aggressively, invade surrounding tissues, and potentially spread to other parts of the body.

Hallmarks of Cancer

Scientists have identified several "hallmarks" of cancer that distinguish cancerous cells from normal cells:

Sustaining Proliferative Signaling:
Cancer cells can continuously signal themselves to grow and divide.

Evading Growth Suppressors: Cancer cells can ignore signals that normally tell cells to stop growing.

Resisting Cell Death: Normal cells undergo programmed cell death (apoptosis) when damaged, but cancer cells can evade this process.

Enabling Replicative Immortality: Cancer cells can divide indefinitely, unlike normal cells that have a limited number of divisions.

Inducing Angiogenesis: Cancer cells can stimulate the formation of new blood vessels to supply the growing tumor with nutrients.

Activating Invasion and Metastasis: Cancer cells can invade surrounding tissues and spread to distant parts of the body.

Conclusion

Cancer is a multifactorial disease that results from a combination of genetic predisposition, environmental exposures, lifestyle factors, and infections. Understanding the mechanisms behind cancer formation is essential for developing effective prevention, diagnosis, and treatment strategies. Although much progress has been made, cancer research continues to evolve as scientists uncover more about the complex processes involved in carcinogenesis.

Foods to Avoid for Cancer Prevention

Processed Meat

Processed meats, which include products like bacon, sausages, hot dogs, ham, and deli meats, have been linked to an increased risk of cancer, particularly colorectal cancer. The World Health Organization (WHO) classifies processed meats as Group 1 carcinogens, meaning there is strong evidence that these foods can cause cancer in humans.

Types of Processed Meats to Avoid

Bacon

> *Risk:* Contains nitrites and nitrates, which can form carcinogenic compounds called nitrosamines during cooking, especially at high temperatures.

Sausages

> *Risk:* Often contain preservatives, additives, and nitrites. High consumption has been linked to an increased risk of colorectal cancer.

Hot Dogs

> *Risk:* Processed using similar methods as other processed meats, hot dogs are high in sodium and preservatives, contributing to cancer risk.

Ham

> *Risk:* Typically cured with nitrites, which are linked to cancer risk. Smoked and salted varieties pose additional risks due to the presence of carcinogenic compounds formed during processing.

Deli Meats (Cold Cuts)

Risk: Frequently preserved with nitrites and other chemicals, which can contribute to an increased risk of colorectal cancer.

Why These Meats Are Harmful

Nitrites and Nitrates: These preservatives can convert into nitrosamines, potent carcinogens, particularly when meats are cooked at high temperatures.

High Heat Cooking: Cooking processed meats at high temperatures, such as grilling or frying, can lead to the formation of heterocyclic amines (HCAs) and polycyclic aromatic hydrocarbons (PAHs), both of which are carcinogenic.

Sodium Content: Processed meats are often high in sodium, which has been linked to increased risk of stomach cancer.

Chemical Additives: Many processed meats contain additives and preservatives that can have harmful effects on health, including contributing to cancer risk.

Recommendations

To reduce cancer risk, it's advisable to limit or avoid processed meats and opt for healthier protein sources such as:
Lean meats
Legumes
Quinoa
Poultry
Eggs
Fish

Plant-based proteins

Focusing on a diet rich in whole foods, such as fruits, vegetables, whole grains, and lean proteins, can help reduce the risk of cancer and promote overall health.

Conclusion

Avoiding processed meats such as hot dogs, ham, and deli meats is a critical step in cancer prevention. These meats are classified as carcinogenic due to their content of harmful substances like nitrites, nitrates, and chemical additives, which can convert into carcinogenic compounds during processing and cooking. High consumption of processed meats is strongly linked to an increased risk of colorectal cancer, among others.

Highly Processed Foods

Highly processed foods, also known as ultra-processed foods, are items that have undergone extensive industrial processing and have multiple ingredients, including preservatives, artificial flavors, colors, and other additives. These foods are often high in sugar, unhealthy fats, and salt, while being low in essential nutrients like fiber, vitamins, and minerals.

Examples of Highly Processed Foods

- *Packaged Snacks:* Chips, cookies, and crackers.
- *Ready-to-Eat Meals:* Frozen dinners, instant noodles, and canned soups.
- *Sugary Cereals:* Breakfast cereals with added sugars and artificial flavors.
- *Processed Meats:* Hot dogs, sausages, and deli meats.
- *Soft Drinks and Sugary Beverages:* Sodas, energy drinks, and sweetened fruit juices.
- *Fast Food:* Burgers, fries, and fried chicken from fast food chains.

Why Avoid Highly Processed Foods for Cancer Prevention?

High in Harmful Additives

Many highly processed foods have artificial preservatives, colorings, and flavorings that have been linked to health issues, including cancer. For example, some studies suggest that certain preservatives and food colorings might have carcinogenic properties or promote the growth of cancer cells.

Excessive Sugar Content

Highly processed foods often have large amounts of added sugars, which can lead to obesity—a known risk factor for several types of cancer, including breast, colorectal, and pancreatic cancer. High sugar intake can also cause chronic inflammation and insulin resistance, both of which may contribute to cancer development.

Unhealthy Fats

These foods are often high in unhealthy fats, particularly trans fats and saturated fats. Diets high in these fats have been associated with an increased risk of cancer, particularly breast and colorectal cancers. Trans fats can promote inflammation, which is a risk factor for cancer.

Low Nutritional Value

Highly processed foods are typically low in essential nutrients such as fiber, vitamins, and antioxidants that help protect against cancer. A diet lacking in these nutrients can weaken the body's defense mechanisms against oxidative stress and inflammation, which are key factors in cancer development.

Promoting Obesity

The high calorie density and low satiety value of ultra-processed foods can contribute to overeating and weight gain, leading to obesity. Obesity is a significant risk factor for many cancers, including endometrial, esophageal, and kidney cancers.

Chemical Contaminants

During the processing of these foods, harmful chemicals like acrylamide (formed during high-temperature cooking processes like frying) and nitrosamines (found in processed meats) can be produced. These chemicals have been identified as potential carcinogens.

Supporting Studies and Evidence

World Health Organization (WHO) and International Agency for Research on Cancer (IARC): Both organizations have classified processed meats as carcinogenic to humans, linking them to colorectal cancer. These findings extend concerns to other highly processed foods, which may contain similar harmful compounds.

American Cancer Society: Recommends a diet rich in fruits, vegetables, and whole grains while limiting the intake of processed and red meats, sugary drinks, and highly processed foods to reduce cancer risk.

Recent Research: A 2018 study published in the *BMJ* found that a 10% increase in the consumption of ultra-processed foods was associated with a 12% increase in the risk of overall cancer and an 11% increase in the risk of breast cancer.

Conclusion

Avoiding or significantly reducing the intake of highly processed foods can be an important step in cancer prevention. Instead, focus on a diet rich in whole, minimally processed foods like fruits, vegetables, whole grains, lean proteins, and healthy fats, which provide essential nutrients and protect against cancer.

Seed and Vegetable Oils

Seed oils and vegetable oils, such as soybean oil, corn oil, sunflower oil, and canola oil, are prevalent in many diets but pose certain health risks. Here is a detailed look at the potential negatives of these oils, particularly how the body processes them, their link to free radicals, and their association with cancer:

High Omega-6 Fatty Acid Content:

Seed and vegetable oils are high in omega-6 polyunsaturated fatty acids (PUFAs). While omega-6 fats are essential, an excessive intake relative to omega-3 fatty acids can lead to chronic inflammation.

The typical Western diet often has a high omega-6 to omega-3 ratio, which is linked to increased inflammation, a risk factor for many chronic diseases, including cancer.

Oxidation and Free Radical Formation:

Omega-6 fatty acids are prone to oxidation, especially when exposed to heat, light, or air. This oxidation leads to the production of harmful compounds like lipid peroxides and aldehydes.

These oxidized compounds can damage cells and tissues, contributing to oxidative stress. Oxidative stress is a known factor in the development of chronic diseases, including cancer.

Impact on Cell Membranes:

The fatty acids we consume are incorporated into our cell membranes. A diet high in omega-6 fatty acids can alter the fatty acid composition of cell membranes, making them more susceptible to oxidative damage.

This oxidative damage to cell membranes can affect cell signaling and function, potentially leading to the development of cancerous cells.

Promotion of Inflammatory Pathways:

Omega-6 fatty acids are precursors to pro-inflammatory molecules called eicosanoids. Elevated levels of these inflammatory mediators can promote an environment conducive to cancer development and progression.

Processed and Refined Oils:

Many seed and vegetable oils are highly processed and refined. The refining process often involves high heat and chemical treatments, which can further promote the formation of harmful oxidation products.

These refined oils may also contain residues from the chemical processing methods, contributing to additional health risks.

Link to Cancer

Inflammation and Cancer:

Chronic inflammation is a well-established risk factor for cancer. Inflammatory processes can lead to DNA damage, promote tumor growth, and facilitate the spread of cancer cells.

By contributing to systemic inflammation, high consumption of omega-6 fatty acids from seed and vegetable oils may increase cancer risk.

Oxidative Stress and DNA Damage:

Oxidative stress resulting from the consumption of oxidized omega-6 fatty acids can damage DNA, proteins, and cellular structures. DNA damage is a critical step in the initiation and progression of cancer.

Free radicals and oxidative stress can also activate signaling pathways that promote cell proliferation and survival, further contributing to cancer development.

Dietary Imbalance:

The imbalance between omega-6 and omega-3 fatty acids in the diet can disrupt normal cellular functions and promote an environment conducive to cancer.

A diet that minimizes the intake of omega-6-rich seed and vegetable oils while emphasizing omega-3 sources (such as fish, flaxseeds, and chia seeds) will help reduce inflammation and oxidative stress, lowering cancer risk.

Recommendations for Healthier Oils

To promote better health and reduce the potential risks associated with seed and vegetable oils, consider the following alternatives:

Olive Oil: Rich in monounsaturated fats and antioxidants, olive oil is a healthier choice for cooking and salad dressings.

Coconut Oil: Contains medium-chain triglycerides (MCTs) that are more stable and less prone to oxidation compared to polyunsaturated fats.

Avocado Oil: High in monounsaturated fats and stable at hot temperatures, making it suitable for cooking.

Butter and Ghee: Natural sources of saturated fats that are stable for cooking and free from harmful processing chemicals.

Conclusion

The consumption of seed and vegetable oils high in omega-6 fatty acids, such as soybean, corn, sunflower, and canola oil, poses potential health risks due to their contribution to chronic inflammation, oxidative stress, and DNA damage—factors linked to cancer development. These oils are prone to oxidation, especially when exposed to heat, leading to the formation of harmful compounds like lipid peroxides and aldehydes, which can damage cells and promote inflammatory pathways. Additionally, the dietary imbalance between omega-6 and omega-3 fatty acids, common in the Western diet, further worsens these risks.

To reduce the potential health hazards associated with these oils, it's advisable to minimize their intake and opt for healthier alternatives. Oils such as olive oil, coconut oil, avocado oil, and natural sources like butter and ghee are more stable and less likely to contribute to inflammation and oxidative stress. By choosing these alternatives, you can promote better overall health and potentially reduce your risk of cancer.

Artificial Sweeteners

Artificial sweeteners are synthetic sugar substitutes often used to reduce calorie intake. While they are approved for use by regulatory agencies like the FDA, there is ongoing debate about their long-term health effects, including potential links to cancer. Here's a look at some artificial sweeteners you might consider avoiding for cancer prevention:

Aspartame

Where it is found: Diet sodas, sugar-free gum, sugar-free desserts, and tabletop sweeteners like Equal and NutraSweet.

Health Concerns: Aspartame has been one of the most extensively studied artificial sweeteners. Some studies in animals have suggested a potential link between aspartame and cancer, particularly brain cancer and leukemia. However, studies in humans have not conclusively proven this connection. Despite this, concerns about its safety persist, leading some health advocates to recommend caution.

Saccharin

Where it is found: Sweet' N Low, diet soft drinks, and low-calorie foods.

Health Concerns: Saccharin was once linked to bladder cancer in laboratory rats, leading to its inclusion on a list of potential carcinogens. However, later studies in humans did not show the same risk, and it was removed from the list in the U.S. in 2000. Despite this, the historical concerns still lead some to avoid saccharin as a precaution.

Sucralose

Where it is found: Splenda, baked goods, and beverages.

Health Concerns: Sucralose is considered safe, but there have been some studies that raise concerns about its effects when heated. For example, sucralose can break down at high temperatures, potentially releasing harmful compounds. Although there is no convincing evidence linking sucralose to cancer, its breakdown products are still under investigation.

Acesulfame Potassium (Acesulfame K)

Where it is found: Sugar-free products like gum, baked goods, and diet sodas.

Health Concerns: Acesulfame K has been criticized for its potential to cause cancer. Some studies in animals have suggested that it might affect DNA, leading to cancer, although these findings are not confirmed in humans. The sweetener contains methylene chloride, a known carcinogen, although the levels in Acesulfame K are considered safe by regulatory bodies. A recent study from the NutriNet-Santé project, which tracked over 100,000 French participants, found that high consumption of aspartame and acesulfame-K was associated with a higher risk of breast and obesity-related cancers. Participants consuming the most artificial sweeteners had a 13% increased risk of developing cancer compared to those who consumed none. A study by the Ramazzini Institute confirmed that aspartame, a widely used artificial sweetener, is a chemical carcinogen in rodents. The study found that aspartame causes malignant tumors in multiple organs, with prenatal exposure increasing cancer risk in offspring even at low doses. This re-evaluation involved immunohistochemical analysis and morphological reassessment, which validated the original findings and refuted claims that the observed tumors were due to infections. These results highlight the need for public health agencies to reassess aspartame's Acceptable Daily Intake (ADI) levels to better protect against cancer risks, especially for vulnerable populations such as pregnant women and children.

Conclusion

Given the potential risks and the ongoing debate over its safety, avoiding Acesulfame potassium could be a cautious choice, particularly for those concerned about cancer prevention. While more research is needed to fully understand the long-term effects of Acesulfame K, opting for natural sweeteners, or reducing overall sweetener intake may be a safer approach.

Sugar

Insulin and Insulin-like Growth Factor (IGF)

Mechanism: High sugar intake can lead to elevated blood glucose levels, which in turn stimulates the production of insulin and IGF. Both insulin and IGF can promote cell proliferation and inhibit apoptosis (programmed cell death), potentially contributing to cancer growth.

Evidence: Elevated levels of insulin and IGF have been associated with an increased risk of various cancers, including breast, colorectal, and prostate cancer.

Obesity and Inflammation

Mechanism: Excessive sugar consumption contributes to obesity, which is a known risk factor for several types of cancer. Obesity leads to chronic low-grade inflammation, which can create an environment conducive to cancer development.

Evidence: Studies have shown that obesity and associated inflammation can promote tumorigenesis (the formation of tumors) and cancer progression.

Increased Cellular Proliferation

Mechanism: Sugars, particularly refined ones, can provide a rapid source of energy for rapidly dividing cancer cells. High sugar levels might support the growth and spread of existing tumors.

Evidence: Cancer cells often exhibit high rates of glucose uptake and metabolism (known as the Warburg effect), which supports their rapid proliferation.

Glycemic Index and Load

Mechanism: Foods with a high glycemic index (GI) and glycemic load (GL) cause quick spikes in blood glucose and insulin levels.

Frequent consumption of high-GI foods can lead to chronic hyperglycemia and hyperinsulinemia, potentially increasing cancer risk.

Evidence: Diets high in GI and GL have been associated with a higher risk of certain cancers, though the exact relationship can vary by cancer type.

Research Findings

Epidemiological Studies

Findings: Observational studies have found associations between high sugar intake and increased cancer risk. For example, higher consumption of sugary beverages has been linked to a greater risk of obesity-related cancers.

Animal Studies

Findings: Research in animal models has shown that high sugar diets can accelerate tumor growth and metastasis. However, translating these findings to humans requires further investigation.

Conclusion

Excessive sugar consumption is linked to various mechanisms that could potentially contribute to cancer development and progression, including insulin resistance, obesity, and increased cellular proliferation. While the evidence suggests that high sugar intake may increase cancer risk, particularly through indirect pathways like obesity and inflammation, more research is needed to clarify the direct effects of sugar on cancer.

Healthy Alternatives to Processed Sugars

While it is crucial to avoid harmful sweeteners, it is equally important to know about healthier alternatives. Here are some natural sweeteners that can be used as part of a balanced diet:

Monk Fruit:

A natural sweetener derived from monk fruit, it contains zero calories and has a glycemic index of zero, making it a safe option for diabetics and those looking to reduce sugar intake.

Honey:

While higher in calories, honey has antioxidant properties and can be used in moderation as a natural sweetener.

Maple Syrup:

A natural sweetener that contains beneficial minerals and antioxidants. It should be used sparingly due to its high sugar content.

Coconut Sugar:

Made from the sap of coconut palm trees, it has a lower glycemic index than regular sugar and retains some nutrients found in the coconut palm.

Fruit Sugars (Fructose):

Natural sugars found in fruits are accompanied by fiber, vitamins, and minerals, making them a healthier option compared to processed sugars.

Natural Sweeteners:

Studies in "Nutrients" highlight the benefits of monk fruit and stevia as safe alternatives with minimal health risks.

Conclusion

Adopting a diet rich in natural, unprocessed foods can play a crucial role in cancer prevention. The principle is simple: if it comes from nature and remains unaltered, it is beneficial. Conversely, foods that are highly processed or extracted often lose their nutritional value and may even become harmful. All things in moderation of course.

Anti-Cancer Foods

Many foods have been studied for their potential cancer-fighting properties due to their nutrient content and bioactive compounds. Here is a list of some notable anti-cancer foods along with the scientific evidence supporting their benefits:

Berries:

Types: Blueberries, strawberries, raspberries, blackberries.

Benefits: Berries are rich in antioxidants, such as vitamins C and E, and phytochemicals like flavonoids and anthocyanins.

Evidence: Studies have shown that the antioxidants in berries can help protect cells from damage caused by free radicals, potentially reducing the risk of cancer. Some studies also suggest that compounds in berries may inhibit the growth of cancer cells and reduce inflammation.

Leafy Greens:

Types: Spinach, kale, Swiss chard, arugula.

Benefits: Leafy greens are high in vitamins (A, C, K), minerals (calcium, iron), and fiber, and contain antioxidants and phytochemicals such as lutein and zeaxanthin.

Evidence: Consumption of leafy greens has been linked to a lower risk of certain cancers, such as breast and colorectal cancer, due to their nutrient density and ability to support detoxification processes in the body.

Cruciferous Vegetables:

Types: Broccoli, cauliflower, Brussels sprouts, cabbage.

Benefits: These vegetables contain glucosinolates, which are sulfur-containing compounds that can form biologically active compounds like indoles and isothiocyanates.

Evidence: These compounds have been shown to inhibit the development and progression of cancer by protecting cells from DNA damage, inactivating carcinogens, and inducing apoptosis (programmed cell death).

Garlic and Onions:

Benefits: Contain organosulfur compounds, which have been found to have anti-cancer effects.

Evidence: Studies suggest that these compounds may help reduce the risk of cancer by detoxifying carcinogens, reducing inflammation, and inhibiting cancer cell growth and metastasis.

Nuts and Seeds:

Types: Walnuts, almonds, flaxseeds, chia seeds.

Benefits: High in healthy fats, fiber, vitamins, minerals, and antioxidants.

Evidence: Regular consumption of nuts and seeds has been associated with a reduced risk of certain cancers, including breast and colorectal cancer, due to their ability to reduce inflammation, oxidative stress, and improve gut health.

Green Tea:

Benefits: Rich in polyphenols, particularly catechins like epigallocatechin-3-gallate (EGCG).

Evidence: Green tea polyphenols have been shown to have antioxidant properties, inhibit tumor cell proliferation, and induce apoptosis in cancer cells. Some epidemiological studies suggest that regular green tea consumption is associated with a reduced risk of certain cancers.

Tomatoes:

Benefits: High in lycopene, a powerful antioxidant.

Evidence: Lycopene has been shown to protect against certain types of cancer, particularly prostate cancer. Cooking tomatoes increases the bioavailability of lycopene, making tomato-based sauces particularly beneficial.

Turmeric:

Benefits: Contains curcumin, which has potent anti-inflammatory and antioxidant properties.

Evidence: Curcumin has been extensively studied for its potential to inhibit cancer cell growth, induce apoptosis, and prevent metastasis. It has shown promise in the treatment and prevention of various cancers in laboratory and animal studies.

Beans and Legumes

Benefit: These foods are rich in essential nutrients such as folate, iron, potassium, and magnesium, which contribute to overall health and can have protective effects against cancer.

Evidence: Micronutrients like folate are involved in DNA repair and synthesis, potentially reducing cancer risk.

Anti-Cancer Diet

Creating a balanced anti-cancer diet involves incorporating a variety of nutrient-dense foods that have been shown to have cancer-fighting properties. Here are some nutritional guidelines, meal planning tips, and sample meal plans with recipes to help you get started:

Nutritional Guidelines

Eat a Variety of Fruits and Vegetables:

- Aim for at least 5 servings of fruits and vegetables daily.
- Include a variety of colors to ensure a range of nutrients and phytochemicals.

Choose Whole Grains:

- Replace refined grains with whole grains like brown rice, quinoa, barley, and whole wheat.

Incorporate Lean Proteins:

- Include plant-based proteins like beans, lentils, and tofu.
- Choose lean animal proteins such as chicken, turkey, and fish.

Include Healthy Fats:

- Focus on sources of healthy fats like avocados, nuts, seeds, and olive oil.
- Limit saturated fats and avoid trans fats.

Stay Hydrated:

- Drink plenty of water throughout the day.
- Limit sugary drinks and opt for herbal teas or infused water for variety.

Limit Processed Meats:

- Avoid processed meats like sausages, and deli meats.

Reduce Sugar:

- Minimize added sugars in your diet.
- Use herbs and spices to enhance flavor instead.

The Use of Pesticides and the Link to Cancer: An In-Depth Analysis

Introduction

Pesticides are widely used in agriculture to protect crops from pests and diseases, ensuring high yields and stable food supplies. However, their extensive use has raised significant public health concerns, particularly on their potential link to cancer. This article explores the relationship between pesticide exposure and cancer risk, examining scientific evidence, types of pesticides, and their health impacts.

Evidence Linking Pesticides to Cancer

Numerous studies have investigated the potential carcinogenic effects of pesticides. Key findings include:

Epidemiological Studies:

A study published in the *International Journal of Cancer* found that agricultural workers exposed to certain pesticides had a higher incidence of cancers, including non-Hodgkin lymphoma (NHL), leukemia, and prostate cancer. The Agricultural Health Study, a large cohort study, also reported associations between pesticide exposure and various cancers among farmers and their families.

Laboratory Studies:

Animal studies have shown that exposure to certain pesticides can induce tumors in rodents. For instance, organophosphates, a common class of insecticides, have been linked to liver and lung cancers in animal models.

Cell culture studies:

Have proven that some pesticides can cause DNA damage, disrupt endocrine function, and promote oxidative stress, all of which are mechanisms involved in carcinogenesis.

Specific Pesticides and Associated Cancer Risks

Glyphosate:

Glyphosate, the active ingredient in the herbicide Roundup, has been classified by the International Agency for Research on Cancer (IARC) as "probably carcinogenic to humans" (Group 2A). Studies have linked glyphosate exposure to an increased risk of NHL.

Organochlorines:

Pesticides like DDT and chlordane, which are now banned or restricted in many countries, have been linked to breast cancer, liver cancer, and NHL. These chemicals persist in the environment and accumulate in the food chain, posing long-term health risks.

Carbamates and Organophosphates:

These insecticides have been associated with increased risks of leukemia, lymphoma, and brain cancer. Their potential to cause cancer is believed to stem from their ability to induce genetic mutations and disrupt hormonal balance.

Conclusion

The link between pesticide exposure and cancer is supported by substantial scientific evidence, highlighting the need for cautious use and stringent regulation of these chemicals. While pesticides play a crucial role in modern agriculture, their potential health risks cannot be ignored. Continued research, along with improved regulatory measures, is essential to protect public health while ensuring agricultural productivity. Consumers can also mitigate risks by choosing organic produce, thoroughly washing fruits and vegetables, and advocating for safer pest control methods.

Natural Remedies with Conventional Treatments

Fenbendazole

An antiparasitic drug commonly used to treat parasitic infections in animals, has recently gained attention for its potential use in cancer treatment. Here is a detailed overview of the current understanding of fenbendazole and its implications for cancer treatment.

What is Fenbendazole?

While fenbendazole's primary use is in veterinary medicine, its potential anti-cancer properties have sparked interest in the medical community. Let's explore the mechanisms by which this compound may affect cancer cells.

Classification:

- Fenbendazole is a benzimidazole carbamate, an anthelmintic drug used to treat infections caused by gastrointestinal parasites such as roundworms, hookworms, and tapeworms in animals.

Mechanism of Action:

- It works by inhibiting microtubule polymerization, which disrupts the cellular structure and function of parasites, leading to their death.

Potential Anti-Cancer Mechanisms

These potential mechanisms of action are intriguing, but how does fenbendazole perform in actual studies? Let us examine the current research evidence.

Disruption of Microtubules:

Cancer Cells: Like its action on parasites, fenbendazole disrupts the microtubule dynamics in cancer cells. Microtubules are essential for cell division, and their disruption can inhibit cancer cell proliferation and induce apoptosis (programmed cell death).

Interference with Glucose Metabolism:

Cancer Metabolism: Cancer cells rely heavily on glycolysis for energy production, even in the presence of oxygen (the Warburg effect). Fenbendazole has been shown to inhibit glucose uptake in cancer cells, thereby starving them of energy and reducing their growth and survival.

Induction of Oxidative Stress:

Reactive Oxygen Species (ROS): Fenbendazole can increase the production of reactive oxygen species in cancer cells. Elevated ROS levels can cause oxidative damage to cellular components, leading to cell death.

Evidence from Research

Despite these promising results in laboratory and animal studies, it is crucial to understand how the broader medical community views fenbendazole as a potential cancer treatment.

Preclinical Studies:

In Vitro Studies: Laboratory studies using cancer cell lines have proven that fenbendazole can inhibit cancer cell growth and induce apoptosis. These studies suggest potential efficacy across diverse types of cancer cells, including colorectal, lung, and prostate cancer cells.

Animal Studies: In vivo studies in animal models have shown that fenbendazole can reduce tumor growth. For instance, a study published in *Scientific Reports* (2018) reported that fenbendazole significantly inhibited tumor growth in a mouse model of metastatic cancer.

Case Reports and Anecdotal Evidence:

Patient Reports: There are reports and case studies of cancer patients experiencing significant improvements or remission after incorporating fenbendazole into their treatment regimen. However, these reports are not scientifically validated and should be interpreted with caution.

Current Position of Medical Community

Given the complex landscape of fenbendazole research and medical opinion, what can we conclude about its potential role in cancer treatment?

Caution Advised: The medical community advises caution due to the lack of robust clinical evidence. Patients are encouraged to consult their healthcare providers before considering fenbendazole as a treatment option.

Need for Research: More research, including controlled clinical trials, is needed to determine the safety, optimal dosage, and efficacy of fenbendazole for cancer treatment.

Conclusion

While fenbendazole shows promise as an anti-cancer agent based on preclinical studies and evidence, its use in cancer treatment is not yet supported by rigorous clinical trials. Patients should not self-medicate with fenbendazole but rather discuss potential treatment options with their healthcare providers. Future research may provide clearer insights into the potential role of fenbendazole in cancer therapy.

The recommended dosage of fenbendazole for cancer treatment is not established, as it is primarily an antiparasitic drug used in veterinary medicine. The dosages used for treating animals are not directly transferable to humans, and there is limited clinical data on its use for cancer in humans. However, there are anecdotal guidelines and some case reports that suggest a protocol for off-label use.

Commonly Cited Dosage for Cancer Treatment (Anecdotal)

While clinical dosage guidelines for fenbendazole in cancer treatment are not established, some protocols have emerged from anecdotal use. It is important to note that these are not officially recommended dosages.

Joe Tippens new and improved protocol

- Fenbendazole (300 mg, 6 days a week) or in the case of severe turbo cancers up to 1 gram.
- Ivermectin (24 mg, 7 days a week) or in the case of severe turbo cancers up to 1mg/kg/day.
- Removing sugar from one's diet is crucial during this protocol. (BMJ 2023)
- Avoid processed foods. (BMJ 2024)
- Bio-Available Curcumin (600mg per day, 2 pills per day 7 days a week).
- Vitamin D (62.5 mcg [2500 IU] seven days a week).
- Tocotrienol and Tocopherol forms (all 8) of Vitamin E (400-800mg per day, 7 days a week). A product called Gamma E by Life Extension.
- CBD oil (1-2 droppers full [equal to 167 to 334 mg per day] under the tongue, 7 days a week) CBD-X: The most potent full spectrum organic CBD oil, with 5,000 milligrams of activated cannabinoids and hemp compounds CBD, CBN & CBG per serving.

Important Considerations

Consultation with a Healthcare Provider:

Before starting any off-label treatment, it is crucial to consult with a healthcare provider. They can provide guidance based on individual health conditions, potential drug interactions, and monitor for adverse effects.

Monitoring for Side Effects:

Potential side effects can include gastrointestinal upset, liver enzyme elevation, and allergic reactions. Regular monitoring by a healthcare provider is recommended.

Quality and Source of Fenbendazole:

Ensure that fenbendazole is obtained from a reliable source and is of pharmaceutical grade. Veterinary formulations are not subject to the same regulatory standards as human medications.

Testimonies of Fenbendazole

To provide a more personal perspective on fenbendazole use, let us examine some patient testimonials. However, it is crucial to remember that these are individual experiences and not scientifically verified outcomes.

Joe Tippens

Background: Joe Tippens was diagnosed with small cell lung cancer in 2016 and was given a few months to live. After hearing about the potential anti-cancer effects of fenbendazole, he decided to incorporate it into his treatment regimen.

Experience: "When I was diagnosed with small cell lung cancer" I was given just a few months to live. Desperate for a solution, I came across research suggesting that fenbendazole, a dog dewormer, could have anti-cancer properties. I decided to try it along with CBD oil, curcumin, and vitamin E. I followed a regimen of taking fenbendazole for three consecutive days, followed by four days off. To my astonishment, my scans started showing significant improvements. My oncologist was skeptical but could not deny the results. Now, years later, I remain cancer-free and continue to take fenbendazole as a precautionary measure. I believe this protocol saved my life."

Christyne Stephens

Background: Diagnosed with stage 4 breast cancer in Oct. 2019

Experience: "I had one chemo session in November and ended up in the hospital with multiple major infections. I decided that chemo was no longer an option. I had a couple of friends mention some natural supplements including high dose melatonin and fenbendazole. Today I got the results of my latest signature test. it was finally negative no sign of cancer DNA in my blood!"

Laurice Panzella

Background: Her husband had Lymphoma

Experience: "I Started my husband on Fenbendazole about 4–5 months after diagnosis. We had already been using other supplemental alternatives, tea, etc. When I came across joe's story. I made sure he started after an MRI. Sure enough, his doctor knew we were using alternatives and said, "what kind of black magic are you using"? LOl I told her, and she was impressed. He did 6 rounds of chemo initially but stopped due to liver and kidney damage with no change in lesions. He has continued fenben twice a day and his most recent scan was NED"!

H. B

Background: Dad diagnosed with liver cancer for the 3rd time in January of 2023 (12 tumors on the liver)

Experience: "This time was more severe vs 2018 and 2021. It has been doing the Joe Tippens Protocall since September 2023 after being told it had progressed to stage 4. Pet scan today, NO ACTIVE CANCER, Dr baffled of course. (Has been on immunotherapy since March 2023, was told it should control the cancer but not cure it.) Praise GOD and thank you to Joe Tippen for sharing his testimony! "

Jane M.

Background: Jane M. had breast cancer and started using fenbendazole as an adjunct therapy.

Experience: "Diagnosed with breast cancer, I underwent the usual treatments but wanted to do more to ensure the cancer didn't return. I learned about fenbendazole and its potential benefits from an online support group. I started taking it along with my usual supplements and noticed an improvement in my overall well-being. My follow-up scans have been clear, and my oncologist has been supportive of my decision to include fenbendazole in my regimen. While I can't definitively say it cured my cancer, I believe it has helped in my journey to stay cancer-free."

Fenbendazole successfully works on multiple cancer types. There are written testimonials on these types of cancers on onedaymd.com

1. Breast Cancer Success Stories
2. Bladder Cancer Success Stories
3. Colon Cancer
4. Kidney Cancer Case Series
5. Liver Cancer
6. Lung Cancer
7. Lymphoma
8. Multiple Myeloma
9. Oral Cancer
10. Pancreatic Cancer
11. Prostate Cancer
12. Sarcoma

13. Squamous Cell Carcinoma
14. Skin Cancer
15. Throat Cancer
16. Thymus cancer
17. Uterine cancer

Ivermectin

Ivermectin is primarily known as an antiparasitic medication, widely used for treating infections caused by various parasites. In recent years, some studies have explored its potential anti-cancer properties. Here is a summary of what is known about ivermectin and its role in cancer treatment:

Mechanisms of Action

Cell Cycle Arrest: Ivermectin has been shown to induce cell cycle arrest in cancer cells, which can inhibit their proliferation.

Apoptosis Induction: Some studies suggest that ivermectin can induce apoptosis (programmed cell death) in cancer cells.

Inhibition of Angiogenesis: Ivermectin may inhibit angiogenesis (the formation of new blood vessels), which is crucial for tumor growth and metastasis.

Interference with Cancer Cell Metabolism: Ivermectin has been reported to interfere with the metabolic pathways of cancer cells, leading to their death.

Research and Studies

In Vitro Studies: Laboratory studies have shown that ivermectin can inhibit the growth of various cancer cell lines, including breast cancer, prostate cancer, and leukemia.

Animal Studies: Some animal studies have demonstrated that ivermectin can reduce tumor growth and improve survival rates in mice with certain types of cancer.

Clinical Trials: As of now, there are limited clinical trials investigating the efficacy and safety of ivermectin in cancer patients. The results of these trials will be crucial to determining its potential as a cancer treatment.

Challenges and Considerations

Dosage and Safety: The doses of ivermectin used in anti-cancer studies are often much higher than those used for antiparasitic treatments. The safety and potential side effects of such high doses need thorough evaluation.

Mechanisms Not Fully Understood: While some mechanisms of action have been proposed, the exact ways in which ivermectin may affect cancer cells are not fully understood.

Combination Therapies: Research is ongoing to see if ivermectin can be used in combination with other cancer treatments to enhance efficacy.

Current Consensus

While preliminary research is promising, ivermectin is not currently approved as a cancer treatment by major health authorities such as the FDA or EMA. More extensive clinical trials are needed to confirm its safety and efficacy in cancer patients.

Conclusion

Ivermectin has shown potential in laboratory and animal studies as an anti-cancer agent, but it is not yet a recognized or approved treatment for cancer in humans. Ongoing research and clinical trials will be essential to determine whether it can be a viable option for cancer therapy in the future.

Ivermectin is a well-established antiparasitic medication, and its dosing varies depending on the type of parasitic infection being treated. Here are the recommended doses for some common parasitic infections:

General Dosage Information

Formulation: Ivermectin is usually available in tablet form.
Administration: It is typically taken on an empty stomach with water.

Common Doses for Specific Conditions

Strongyloidiasis (Intestinal Threadworm)

> *Adults and Children:* The typical dose is 200 micrograms per kilogram (mcg/kg) of body weight as a single dose.
> *Example:* For a 70 kg adult, the dose would be 14 mg (200 mcg/kg × 70 kg = 14,000 mcg or 14 mg).

Onchocerciasis (River Blindness)

> *Adults and Children:* The recommended dose is 150 mcg/kg of body weight, taken as a single dose.
> *Example:* For a 70 kg adult, the dose would be 10.5 mg (150 mcg/kg × 70 kg = 10,500 mcg or 10.5 mg).

Lice and Scabies

> *Lice:* A single dose of 200 mcg/kg, with a repeat dose after 7 days if needed.

> *Scabies:* A single dose of 200 mcg/kg, with a repeat dose after 1-2 weeks if needed.

Important Considerations

> *Weight-Based Dosing:* Ivermectin doses are typically calculated based on body weight, so it's important to follow dosing instructions carefully.
> *Medical Supervision:* Always use ivermectin under the guidance of a healthcare professional, especially for conditions requiring multiple doses or for individuals with specific health concerns.

Administration Tips

> *Empty Stomach:* Take ivermectin on an empty stomach, at least 1 hour before or 2 hours after a meal.

> *Hydration:* Drink plenty of water with the medication to ensure proper absorption.

Conclusion

Ivermectin is effective for various parasitic infections when used at the correct dose. Always consult with a healthcare provider for personalized dosing and to ensure safe and effective treatment. Avoid self-medicating and follow professional medical advice for the best outcomes.

Testimonies of ivermectin

Karen

"I was diagnosed with stage IV lung cancer, and after several rounds of chemotherapy, I was feeling defeated. A family member suggested I look into ivermectin after hearing about its potential benefits. I did my own research and decided to incorporate it into my regimen. While I continued my traditional treatments, I felt a renewed sense of hope. I experienced fewer side effects, and my latest scans showed some positive changes. I don't know if it was the ivermectin, but I felt it was worth trying."

David

"When I was diagnosed with liver cancer, I felt overwhelmed. Traditional treatments seemed daunting, so I started exploring alternative options. I came across ivermectin through a support group. I began taking it in conjunction with my prescribed medications. Although I was uncertain about its effectiveness, I felt it helped with my overall energy levels. After a few months, my doctor noted some improvements in my condition. I'm grateful for any support that helped me along the way."

Lisa

"I was looking for anything that could help my situation after being diagnosed with ovarian cancer. I heard about ivermectin from a friend who had success with alternative treatments. I started taking it alongside my chemotherapy. While my doctors were cautious, they allowed me to proceed. I felt a little better during treatment and managed to stay positive throughout my journey. I think every bit of support helped me through this challenging time."

Tom

"After my colorectal cancer diagnosis, I felt desperate for options. I found online discussions about ivermectin and decided to try it after consulting with my naturopath. I combined it with my conventional treatment. While I cannot attribute my recovery solely to ivermectin, it contributed positively to my overall health. I'm now in remission and continuing to explore ways to maintain my health."

Essiac Tea

Essiac tea is an herbal remedy with a long and fascinating history. Developed from an Ojibwa Native American formula and popularized by Canadian nurse Rene Caisse, this blend of four powerful herbs has gained attention for its potential cancer-fighting benefits. While scientific evidence remains limited, Essiac tea is widely used by holistic practitioners and those seeking alternative treatments for cancer due to its detoxifying, immune-boosting, and anti-inflammatory properties.

Essiac tea is typically composed of the following four key ingredients, each with its own therapeutic qualities:

Burdock Root (Arctium lappa)

Known for its detoxifying effects, burdock root is believed to cleanse the blood and support liver function, making it an essential part of Essiac's formulation. Rich in antioxidants, it may help protect cells from damage and has shown some anti-cancer potential in laboratory studies, particularly for slowing the growth of cancer cells.

Sheep Sorrel (Rumex acetosella)

This herb is at the heart of Essiac's reputation for combating cancer. Sheep sorrel is thought to help regenerate cells and has been explored for its tumor-fighting properties, though more research is needed to confirm its effectiveness in humans.

Slippery Elm (Ulmus rubra)

With its soothing effect on the digestive system, slippery elm aids in reducing inflammation and improving nutrient absorption. This is particularly helpful for cancer patients, as improved digestion can aid in overall health and recovery.

Indian Rhubarb Root (Rheum officinale)

Traditionally used in small amounts for its digestive and detoxifying properties, Indian rhubarb root may assist in cleansing the liver and intestines. It contains compounds that act as a gentle laxative, helping to rid the body of toxins, another crucial element of Essiac's potential anti-cancer effects.

Cancer-Fighting Benefits

Many proponents of Essiac tea believe that its combination of detoxification, immune system support, and anti-inflammatory properties makes it a powerful tool in the fight against cancer.

Here's how it may contribute to cancer prevention and treatment:

Detoxification:

The body's natural detoxification processes are crucial for preventing the buildup of toxins that can contribute to cancer. Essiac tea, with its emphasis on supporting liver health, may help flush out harmful substances, making it harder for cancerous cells to thrive.

Immune System Support:

A strong immune system is the body's first line of defense against cancer. The herbs in Essiac, particularly burdock root, are believed to boost immune function, enabling the body to better recognize and destroy abnormal cells before they turn into cancer.

Anti-Inflammatory Effects:

Chronic inflammation is a key factor in the development of many cancers. Essiac tea's anti-inflammatory properties, especially from ingredients like slippery elm, may help reduce this risk and support the body's overall healing process.

Antioxidant Activity:

Free radicals, which are unstable molecules that can damage healthy cells, play a role in cancer development. Essiac tea's herbs are rich in antioxidants, which neutralize free radicals and may reduce the risk of cellular damage.

Scientific Evidence and Safety Considerations

While anecdotal reports of Essiac tea helping cancer patients abound, the scientific community remains divided. Laboratory studies have shown some anti-cancer activity in individual herbs, particularly burdock root and sheep sorrel, but clinical trials in humans are lacking. As such, Essiac tea should be seen as a complementary therapy rather than a stand-alone cancer treatment.

It's important to consult with a healthcare professional before incorporating Essiac tea into your cancer care plan. The tea is generally safe, but some individuals may experience mild side effects, including nausea, diarrhea, or interactions with medications. Indian rhubarb root can act as a laxative, so it's essential to monitor your body's response carefully.

The Holistic Perspective

In the holistic approach to cancer care, Essiac tea represents a blend of ancient wisdom and natural healing. Its ability to support detoxification, reduce inflammation, and bolster the immune system aligns with the principles of natural health that emphasize supporting the body's own healing mechanisms.

Conclusion

Essiac tea has been widely used as a complementary therapy by some cancer patients, especially within alternative and holistic health communities. Developed from a traditional Native American herbal formula, Essiac tea typically includes burdock root, sheep sorrel, slippery elm bark, and Indian rhubarb root. Supporters believe these herbs work together to detoxify the body, boost immune function, and potentially slow cancer cell growth. However, scientific studies on Essiac tea's effectiveness in treating or curing cancer are limited, and the evidence is inconclusive.

Testimonies of Essiac Tea

Julie Y.

Shared her story of incorporating Essiac into her recovery plan after a cancer diagnosis. She believes it helped prevent recurrence, alongside other lifestyle changes such as regular exercise, stress reduction, and avoiding hormone-rich foods. She continues to take the tea as a preventative measure and highly recommends it to others.

Herm B.

Who was diagnosed with stage 4 prostate cancer in 1999, chose not to undergo chemotherapy or radiation after witnessing the effects of these treatments on his wife and daughter, who both passed away from cancer. Instead, he started using Essiac tea in 2000 and has been cancer-free since. Herm credits the tea for his recovery and continues to recommend it to others.

Bill

Diagnosed with stage 3a non-small cell lung cancer, began using Essiac tea during his treatment. He survived far beyond the 10-15 months he was initially given and believed the tea helped him recover and manage his condition. He took six ounces of the tea every morning and reported that it helped him bounce back from the effects of cancer treatments.

Dave

Diagnosed with advanced prostate cancer, saw his PSA levels drop from 234 to 6.51 after incorporating Essiac tea into his regimen. His tumors also significantly reduced in size, and he attributes much of his success to the tea as part of a holistic approach to his treatment.

Jane

Diagnosed with third-stage ovarian cancer in 1993, rejected chemotherapy and instead used Essiac tea as part of her treatment. Thirty years later, she remains cancer-free and credits the tea along with prayers and lifestyle changes, for her survival.

Artemisinin

Derived from the herb Sweet Wormwood (Artemisia annua), it has shown potential in cancer treatment due to its ability to selectively target cancer cells. Here is an overview of its use for cancer and dosage information based on available research and recommendations:

Mechanism of Action

Artemisinin is believed to exert its anti-cancer effects through several mechanisms:

Iron Dependency: Cancer cells typically have higher levels of iron compared to normal cells. Artemisinin interacts with iron to form free radicals within cancer cells, leading to oxidative stress and ultimately cell death.

Selective Toxicity: Artemisinin appears to selectively target cancer cells while sparing normal cells, which contributes to its lower toxicity profile compared to traditional chemotherapy drugs.

Dosage Information

The dosage of artemisinin for cancer treatment varies based on the specific protocol and individual patient factors. Here are some general guidelines and considerations:

Daily Dosage: Typically, artemisinin is administered orally in doses ranging from 400 to 800 milligrams per day. This dosage range has been used in various studies and protocols.

Duration of Treatment: The duration of treatment with artemisinin can vary. Some protocols suggest treatment periods ranging from several weeks to several months, depending on the specific cancer type and individual response.

Combination Therapy: Artemisinin is often used in combination with other supplements or therapies to enhance its efficacy. For example, it may be combined with iron supplements to maximize its cytotoxic effects within cancer cells.

Safety and Monitoring: Artemisinin is generally well-tolerated with minimal side effects reported in clinical studies. However, as with any treatment, it's important to monitor for potential adverse effects and to adjust dosage as needed based on individual response and tolerance.

Practical Considerations

Consultation with Healthcare Provider: It's crucial to consult with a healthcare provider, particularly an oncologist or integrative medicine specialist, before starting artemisinin or any complementary therapy for cancer. They can provide guidance tailored to your specific health status and treatment plan.

Quality and Source: Ensure you obtain artemisinin from a reputable source to ensure purity and quality. Herbal supplements can vary in potency and composition, so quality control is important.

Integration with Conventional Treatment: Artemisinin is often used as a supplementary therapy alongside conventional cancer treatments such as chemotherapy and radiation. It should not replace standard treatments but rather complement them.

Conclusion

Artemisinin shows promise as a complementary therapy in cancer treatment due to its unique mechanism of action and favorable safety profile. However, more rigorous clinical trials are needed to establish its efficacy and safety in treating various types of cancer. If considering artemisinin for cancer treatment, it's essential to do so under the guidance of a healthcare professional to ensure safety, efficacy, and integration with your overall treatment plan.

Testimonies of Artemisinin

Jennifer M.

Experience: "After my breast cancer diagnosis, I underwent surgery and chemotherapy. A friend suggested I look into artemisinin, derived from the sweet wormwood plant, due to its reported anti-cancer properties. I began taking artemisinin supplements daily, starting with a lower dose and gradually increasing it under the guidance of my naturopath. I noticed an improvement in my overall well-being and energy levels. My follow-up scans have shown no signs of recurrence, and I believe that artemisinin along with my conventional treatments and a healthy lifestyle, played a significant role in my recovery."

Robert T.

Experience: "Diagnosed with colorectal cancer, I had surgery and chemotherapy but wanted to leave no stone unturned in my fight against the disease. I read about artemisinin's potential anti-cancer effects and decided to try it. I took 400mg of artemisinin daily, and over time, I felt more energetic and less fatigued from my treatments. My latest scans have shown a significant reduction in tumor size, and my oncologist was pleased with my progress. I believe artemisinin has been a helpful addition to my treatment plan."

Linda S.

Experience: "When I was diagnosed with stage IV lung cancer, I felt devastated and overwhelmed. I started chemotherapy but also researched alternative treatments that could support my recovery. I came across artemisinin and decided to include it in my regimen. I took 600mg of artemisinin daily, along with other supplements and a healthy diet. My energy levels improved, and my side effects from chemotherapy were more manageable. After several months, my scans showed stable disease with no new growth. I believe that artemisinin helped support my body during this challenging time."

Mark D.

Experience: "After being diagnosed with prostate cancer, I opted for surgery followed by radiation therapy. I also wanted to explore natural supplements to aid my recovery. I started taking artemisinin supplements, starting with 200mg and gradually increasing to 600mg daily. I noticed that my recovery from surgery was smoother, and my energy levels were better than expected. My PSA levels have remained low, and my latest biopsy showed no signs of cancer. While I can't say that artemisinin alone cured my cancer, I believe it has been an important part of my holistic approach to treatment."

Rachel K.

Experience: "After my ovarian cancer diagnosis, I underwent surgery and chemotherapy. I read about the potential benefits of artemisinin and decided to try it. I started with 400mg daily and gradually increased the dose. I felt that it helped me cope with the side effects of chemotherapy better and improved my overall sense of well-being. My oncologist was supportive of my decision to include artemisinin in my treatment plan. My recent scans have been clear, and I feel optimistic about the future. I believe that artemisinin has been a valuable part of my recovery process."

Soursop

Also known as graviola or by its scientific name **Annona muricata**, is a tropical fruit that has garnered attention for its potential anti-cancer properties. Here is an overview of soursop and its use in cancer treatment:

Overview of Soursop

Appearance: Soursop is a large, green, spiky fruit with white, fibrous flesh and a unique sweet-sour taste.

Nutritional Content: Rich in vitamins (C, B1, and B2), minerals (magnesium, potassium), and dietary fiber.

Potential Anti-Cancer Properties

Acetogenins:

Soursop contains a class of compounds known as acetogenins. These are considered the primary bioactive components with potential anti-cancer effects.

Mechanism: Acetogenins are thought to inhibit the enzyme complex I of the mitochondrial electron transport chain in cancer cells, leading to decreased ATP production and induction of apoptosis (programmed cell death).

Cytotoxic Activity:

Studies: Several in vitro studies (lab studies using cancer cell lines) have proven that soursop extracts can exert cytotoxic effects on a variety of cancer cells, including breast, prostate, liver, lung, and pancreatic cancer cells.

Selectivity: Some studies suggest that acetogenins may selectively target cancer cells while sparing normal cells, though this selectivity needs further validation.

Anti-Inflammatory and Antioxidant Effects:

Soursop shows anti-inflammatory and antioxidant properties that can contribute to its potential anti-cancer effects. Chronic inflammation and oxidative stress are known to promote cancer development and progression.

Research Evidence

Preclinical Studies:

In Vitro: Numerous laboratory studies have shown that soursop extracts can inhibit the growth and proliferation of various cancer cell lines.

In Vivo: Animal studies have provided some evidence that soursop extracts can reduce tumor size and improve survival rates in cancer models.

Human Studies:

Limited Clinical Trials: As of now, there are very few clinical trials involving humans to conclusively establish the efficacy and safety of soursop for cancer treatment. Most of the evidence is preliminary and derived from cell culture and animal studies.

Potential Risks and Side Effects

Neurotoxicity:

Some studies have suggested that compounds in soursop, particularly annonacin, may have neurotoxic effects, potentially contributing to the development of neuropathies and conditions like Parkinson's disease with prolonged and high-dose use.

Interaction with Conventional Treatments:

Soursop may interact with certain chemotherapy drugs or other medications, potentially affecting their efficacy or causing adverse effects. It is important to discuss with a healthcare provider before using soursop as a complementary treatment.

Current Position in Medical Community

Complementary Treatment: Soursop is sometimes used as a complementary treatment in integrative oncology but not as a standalone cure for cancer. It should be considered as part of a broader treatment plan under the guidance of a healthcare professional.

Need for Further Research: More rigorous clinical trials are needed to determine the efficacy, safety, and appropriate dosage of soursop in cancer treatment.

Recommendations

Consultation: Always consult with a healthcare provider before starting any new treatment, including natural supplements like soursop.

Moderation: If used, soursop should be consumed in moderation, keeping an eye on any potential side effects or interactions with other treatments.

Recommended Dosage of Soursop

The optimal dosage of soursop for its potential health benefits, including its possible anti-cancer properties, is not well-established due to the lack of extensive clinical research. However, general guidelines based on traditional use and preliminary studies can be considered:

Fresh Fruit:

- *Serving Size:* 1 cup (about 150-200 grams) of fresh soursop pulp per day.
- *Frequency:* Up to several times a week.

Soursop Tea:

- *Preparation:* Boil 1-2 soursop leaves in 3 cups of water for 10-15 minutes.
- *Dosage:* Consume 1-2 cups of soursop tea per day.

Soursop Extracts and Supplements:

- *Form:* Capsules, tinctures, or powdered extracts.
- *Dosage:* Follow the manufacturer's instructions, typically ranging from 500 mg to 1500 mg per day.
- *Note:* Consult a healthcare provider before starting any soursop supplements.

Potential Risks and Considerations

Neurotoxicity: Long-term consumption of large amounts of soursop or its extracts has been linked to potential neurotoxic effects, including symptoms similar to Parkinson's disease. Moderation is key.

Interactions: Soursop may interact with certain medications, including blood pressure and diabetes medications. Always consult with a healthcare provider before adding soursop to your diet, especially if you are on medication or have a medical condition.

Pregnancy and Breastfeeding: The safety of soursop during pregnancy and breastfeeding is not well-studied. It's best to avoid or consult a healthcare provider.

Conclusion

Soursop has promising potential health benefits, including anti-cancer properties, but its use should be approached with caution due to the lack of extensive human studies and potential side effects. Moderate consumption of soursop as part of a balanced diet can be beneficial, but it is essential to consult with a healthcare provider before making significant changes to your diet or starting new supplements.

Testimonies of soursop

Karen M.

Experience: "When I was diagnosed with early-stage breast cancer, I was terrified of undergoing surgery and chemotherapy. I researched alternative treatments and came across soursop. I decided to use soursop as my primary treatment. I started drinking fresh soursop juice every day and took soursop leaf tea. I closely monitored my condition with regular check-ups and scans. Over the months, my tumor shrank significantly, and my energy levels improved. My doctor was initially skeptical but couldn't deny the positive changes in my scans. I continue to use soursop daily and remain cancer-free."

Peter R.

Experience: "After being diagnosed with prostate cancer, I was determined to avoid conventional treatments like surgery and radiation. I read about the potential anti-cancer properties of soursop and decided to try it. I started consuming soursop fruit and drinking soursop leaf tea daily. My PSA levels began to drop, and I felt healthier overall. I continued with this regimen, and my latest scans have shown no signs of cancer. I believe that soursop has been instrumental in my recovery, and I am grateful for discovering this natural remedy."

Lisa T.

Experience: "When I was diagnosed with stage II ovarian cancer, I wanted to find a natural approach to treatment. I learned about soursop's potential benefits and decided to use it exclusively. I started drinking soursop leaf tea multiple times a day and ate the fruit whenever I could find it. I focused on maintaining a healthy diet and lifestyle to support my treatment. Over time, my symptoms improved, and my tumor markers decreased. My follow-up scans have been clear, and I believe that soursop has played a crucial role in my recovery."

Michael B.

Experience: "After being diagnosed with colorectal cancer, I was hesitant to undergo chemotherapy and surgery due to the potential side effects. I researched alternative treatments and came across soursop. I decided to use soursop as my sole treatment. I consumed soursop juice daily and took soursop leaf capsules. My overall health improved, and my energy levels increased. My recent scans have shown a reduction in tumor size, and my doctor has been surprised by my progress. I am confident that soursop has been the key to my recovery."

Emily J.

Experience: "When I was diagnosed with lung cancer, I was overwhelmed and scared. I wanted to find a natural treatment option and discovered soursop. I decided to use soursop as my primary treatment. I started drinking soursop leaf tea and consuming the fruit regularly. I also made significant changes to my diet and lifestyle to support my treatment. Over time, my symptoms improved, and my scans showed no new growth. I believe that soursop has been a vital part of my recovery, and I am grateful for its benefits."

Antineoplaston therapy

Is an alternative cancer treatment developed by Dr. Stanislaw Burzynski, a Polish American physician and biochemist. Here is an overview of antineoplaston therapy, its principles, controversies, and status:

Principles of Antineoplaston Therapy

Discovery: Antineoplastons are peptides and amino acid derivatives found in blood and urine. According to Dr. Burzynski, they are naturally occurring substances that control and prevent the growth of cancer cells.

Mechanism of Action: The theory behind antineoplaston therapy posits that cancer results from a deficiency in or lack of normal antineoplaston levels in the body. By providing supplemental antineoplastons, the therapy aims to correct this deficiency and inhibit cancer cell growth while promoting normal cell function and apoptosis (programmed cell death).

Forms of Administration: Antineoplastons can be administered orally or intravenously, depending on the specific formulation and treatment plan prescribed by a licensed physician.

Clinical Applications and Research

Clinical Trials: Dr. Burzynski conducted clinical trials on antineoplaston therapy throughout the 1980s and 1990s. These trials included patients with diverse types of cancer, including brain tumors, lymphoma, and breast cancer.

Results: Some early trials reported promising results, including tumor regression and improved survival rates in certain patients. However, many of these studies were criticized for their design, lack of rigorous controls, and small sample sizes.

Controversies: The efficacy and safety of antineoplaston therapy has been highly controversial within the medical community. Critics argue that:

Lack of Reproducibility: Independent studies have failed to replicate the positive results reported by Dr. Burzynski.

Regulatory Issues: The U.S. Food and Drug Administration (FDA) has issued warnings and taken legal action against Dr. Burzynski for marketing unapproved drugs and conducting clinical trials without adequate oversight.

Ethical Concerns: Questions have been raised about the ethics of charging patients for participation in clinical trials and the scientific validity of the therapy.

Current Status

Legal and Regulatory Status: Antineoplaston therapy is not approved by the FDA or other regulatory agencies as a standard cancer treatment. It is considered an experimental therapy and is typically only available through clinical trials or under compassionate use protocols.

Patient Access: Despite regulatory challenges, some patients continue to seek antineoplaston therapy through Dr. Burzynski's clinic in Texas or other providers offering alternative cancer treatments.

Scientific Community Perspective: The mainstream medical and scientific communities remain skeptical due to the lack of robust clinical evidence supporting the efficacy and safety of antineoplaston therapy. Most oncologists do not recommend it as a primary or supplementary treatment for cancer.

Conclusion

Antineoplaston therapy represents a controversial approach to cancer treatment based on the concept of using peptides and amino acid derivatives to control cancer cell growth. While some early studies showed promising results, the therapy lacks widespread acceptance due to concerns over study design, reproducibility, regulatory issues, and ethical considerations. Patients considering alternative treatments like antineoplaston therapy should consult with qualified healthcare professionals and carefully evaluate the available evidence and risks.

Testimonies Antineoplaston

Laura Hymas

Testimony: "I was diagnosed with Glioblastoma Multiforme in 2011 and was given a poor prognosis. After researching alternative treatments, I decided to pursue antineoplaston therapy at the Burzynski Clinic. The treatment was tough and required commitment, but I started seeing improvements. My tumor shrank significantly, and eventually, I went into remission. I am grateful for the treatment and the support I received from Dr. Burzynski and his team. While it was a challenging journey, I believe antineoplastons played a crucial role in my recovery."

Hannah Bradley

Testimony: "My journey with brain cancer began in 2011, and after conventional treatments failed to provide the results, I hoped for, I learned about antineoplastons. Traveling to Texas for treatment was a big decision, but it offered hope when other options were limited. Over time, I experienced a noticeable reduction in my tumor, and my quality of life improved. The road was not easy, but the therapy provided me with another chance. My family and I remain thankful for the alternative treatment path we chose."

Tori Moreno

Testimony: "When Tori was diagnosed with DIPG, we were devastated by the lack of effective conventional treatments. After extensive research, we decided to try antineoplastons at the Burzynski Clinic. The results were encouraging as Tori showed improvement and had a better quality of life during the treatment. Despite the challenges, we are thankful for the hope and additional time it provided us. Every day with Tori was a blessing, and the treatment offered us precious moments we might not have had otherwise."

Apricot seeds

Specifically, those containing amygdalin (often referred to as vitamin B17 or Laetrile), have been promoted by some as a natural treatment for cancer. Here is an overview of apricot seeds in relation to cancer treatment, including their alleged benefits, potential risks, and current scientific understanding:

Apricot Seeds and Amygdalin (Laetrile)

Source: Apricot seeds contain amygdalin, a plant compound found in the seeds of many fruits, nuts, and plants of the Prunus genus, including apricots, almonds, cherries, and peaches.

Mechanism: Amygdalin is metabolized in the body to release cyanide, which proponents claim selectively targets and kills cancer cells while leaving normal cells unharmed. This concept is based on the idea that cancer cells contain higher levels of beta-glucosidase enzymes, which release cyanide from amygdalin.

Historical Use: Laetrile gained popularity in the 1970s as an alternative cancer treatment, despite limited scientific evidence supporting its efficacy and concerns about toxicity.

Benefits

Anti-Cancer Properties: Advocates claim that amygdalin can kill cancer cells, reduce tumor size, and improve overall health in cancer patients.

Pain Relief: Some anecdotal reports suggest that apricot seeds or amygdalin may alleviate cancer-related pain.

Scientific Perspective

Lack of Evidence: Clinical studies and systematic reviews have not proved conclusive evidence that amygdalin or apricot seeds effectively treat cancer. Most studies have been small, poorly designed, or biased.

Safety Concerns:

Cyanide Toxicity: Amygdalin can release cyanide, which is toxic to humans even in small doses. This toxicity can cause symptoms ranging from dizziness and nausea to more severe neurological and cardiovascular effects.

Lack of Regulation: Dietary supplements containing amygdalin are not regulated by the FDA for safety and efficacy, posing risks of inconsistent dosages and purity.

Legal and Ethical Issues:

Regulatory Actions: The FDA and other health authorities have issued warnings against the use of amygdalin and Laetrile as cancer treatments due to lack of efficacy and potential harm.

False Hope: Using unproven treatments like apricot seeds may lead patients to delay or forego effective conventional therapies, which can impact their prognosis.

Current Recommendations

Medical Community Position: Mainstream medical organizations, including the American Cancer Society and the National Cancer Institute, do not endorse the use of apricot seeds, amygdalin, or Laetrile for cancer treatment due to lack of evidence and safety concerns.

Patient Education: Patients are encouraged to discuss all treatment options with their healthcare providers and to be cautious of alternative therapies that promise miraculous results without scientific support.

Conclusion

While apricot seeds and amygdalin have been promoted as natural cancer treatments, scientific evidence supporting their efficacy and safety is lacking. The potential risks, including cyanide toxicity, outweigh any perceived benefits. Patients diagnosed with cancer should rely on evidence-based treatments recommended by healthcare professionals to optimize their chances of successful outcomes.

Testimonies of Apricot seeds

Sarah J.

> *Testimony:* After being diagnosed with breast cancer, Sarah decided to try a holistic approach in addition to her conventional treatment. She began consuming apricot seeds daily, convinced by the claims of amygdalin's potential anti-cancer effects. Sarah noted a feeling of increased energy and general well-being, and her follow-up scans showed no progression in her cancer. She credits apricot seeds as a vital component of her integrative health routine.

Mark L.

> *Testimony:* Mark was diagnosed with stage 3 lung cancer and was exploring various natural therapies to support his treatment. After reading about the benefits of apricot seeds, he started taking a few seeds each day. He reports that, over time, he felt more energetic and noticed a stabilization in his condition. Mark attributes this partly to the addition of apricot seeds, though he continued with his prescribed treatment as well.

Linda W.

> *Testimony:* Linda was diagnosed with colon cancer and began researching natural cancer-fighting remedies. After discovering apricot seeds, she began consuming them regularly and felt they offered her additional energy and a sense of control over her

health. Although her primary treatment included surgery and chemotherapy, she credits apricot seeds with giving her an extra boost in her recovery.

Daniel K.

Testimony: Daniel, facing a prostate cancer diagnosis, added apricot seeds to his routine after hearing they could inhibit cancer cell growth. He took a small number of seeds daily and claims he noticed improvements in his overall energy and mental clarity. He continued with his standard treatment, and his PSA levels remained stable. Daniel believes that apricot seeds contributed positively to his health.

Maya T.

Testimony: Maya, diagnosed with ovarian cancer, added apricot seeds to her daily diet, feeling hopeful about their reputation for natural cancer support. She consumed a few seeds daily and reported feeling more resilient through her treatment, especially during chemotherapy. While Maya acknowledges her recovery was multifactorial, she believes the apricot seeds supported her immune system and energy levels.

John B.

Testimony: After his pancreatic cancer diagnosis, John researched alternative treatments and came across apricot seeds. He decided to consume a few each day along with his prescribed treatment. John shared that he felt a reduction in his fatigue and attributed some of his resilience to the seeds. His family observed that he seemed more alert and energetic, and he became an advocate for integrating natural therapies.

Vitamin E (Tocotrienols)

Studies on the combination of vitamin E, specifically tocotrienols, with chemotherapy have shown promising results in enhancing treatment efficacy and reducing chemotherapy-related side effects. Tocotrienols are a form of vitamin E that differ from tocopherols in their chemical structure and biological activity.

Enhanced Anti-Cancer Effects:
>Research suggests that tocotrienols possess anti-cancer properties that can complement the effects of chemotherapy drugs. They have been found to inhibit cancer cell growth, induce apoptosis (cell death), and suppress tumor angiogenesis (formation of new blood vessels that support tumor growth).

Protection Against Chemotherapy Toxicity:
>Chemotherapy often causes oxidative stress and damage to healthy cells alongside cancerous ones. Tocotrienols act as antioxidants, scavenging free radicals and reducing oxidative stress. This antioxidant activity may help protect normal cells from chemotherapy-induced damage.

Synergistic Effects:
>Some studies indicate that tocotrienols can synergize with certain chemotherapy drugs to enhance their cytotoxic effects against cancer cells. This synergy potentially allows for lower doses of chemotherapy drugs to be used, minimizing side effects without compromising efficacy.

Reduction of Side Effects:
>One significant benefit of combining tocotrienols with chemotherapy is the potential reduction in side effects commonly associated with chemotherapy, such as nausea, vomiting, fatigue, and hair loss. By protecting healthy cells,

tocotrienols may improve overall patient well-being during treatment.

Clinical Studies and Evidence:

Clinical trials exploring the combination of tocotrienols with chemotherapy are ongoing. Preliminary results from these studies have shown encouraging outcomes, although more extensive research is needed to establish definitive guidelines for clinical use.

Conclusion

While the study of tocotrienols in combination with chemotherapy represents a promising area of research, further clinical trials are necessary to validate these findings and determine optimal treatment protocols. Integrative approaches that combine effective conventional therapies with supportive natural compounds like tocotrienols hold potential for improving cancer treatment outcomes and patient quality of life.

Testimonies of Vitamin E (Tocotrienols)

Pamela N.

Testimony: Pamela was diagnosed with estrogen receptor-positive breast cancer and began researching natural supplements that might support her treatment. She came across tocotrienols and was intrigued by their anti-cancer properties. After incorporating tocotrienol supplements into her daily regimen, she reported a sense of greater well-being and energy. Over time, her follow-up scans showed stable results, and she feels tocotrienols played a role in maintaining her health alongside her treatment.

John K.

Testimony: John, a liver cancer patient, shared his story on an alternative health forum, describing how he started using tocotrienols after reading about their potential benefits for liver health and cancer. He was undergoing conventional treatments and took tocotrienols as a complementary supplement. Over several months, he noted improvements in his liver enzyme levels and overall energy, and his doctors reported that his disease was stable. John attributes part of this stability to the regular use of tocotrienols.

Maria L.

Testimony: Diagnosed with stage 3 ovarian cancer, Maria began a strict regimen including dietary changes, supplements, and integrative therapies. Tocotrienols were a major part of her routine, as she believed their antioxidant and anti-cancer properties could help her body fight the disease. She felt that tocotrienols helped her tolerate chemotherapy better, reducing her fatigue and helping maintain her immune function. Although she completed her treatment, Maria continues to take tocotrienols daily as a preventive measure.

Robert H.

Testimony: Robert was diagnosed with prostate cancer in his mid-60s and sought complementary supplements to support his standard treatment plan. After some research, he decided to include tocotrienols, specifically for their potential role in inhibiting cancer cell growth. He reported feeling more energetic and noted a steady PSA (prostate-specific antigen) level, which his doctors observed was stable. Robert continues to take tocotrienols and believes they play a role in maintaining his overall health.

Emily R.

Testimony: Emily shared her journey on a cancer support forum, explaining how she added tocotrienols to her regimen after her pancreatic cancer diagnosis. Although her prognosis was challenging, she felt that tocotrienols helped reduce some of her chemotherapy side effects, such as inflammation and fatigue. Emily continues to advocate for tocotrienols, stating they provided her with both physical and emotional benefits during her treatment.

James T.

Testimony: James, diagnosed with chronic lymphocytic leukemia (CLL), started researching supplements that could help support his immune system. He began taking tocotrienols after finding studies suggesting benefits for immune health and potential anti-cancer effects. James reports feeling generally healthier and experiencing fewer infections, which he attributes to his regular tocotrienol supplementation.

Turkey Tail Mushroom

Scientifically known as Trametes versicolor or Coriolus versicolor, has gained attention for its potential benefits when used alongside chemotherapy in cancer treatment. Here are some key aspects to consider regarding its effects:

Immune System Support:

Turkey tail mushroom is rich in polysaccharopeptides (PSP) and polysaccharides (beta-glucans) that are believed to stimulate and modulate the immune system. Chemotherapy often suppresses the immune system, making patients more susceptible to infections. Turkey tail mushroom may help strengthen immune function, potentially reducing the risk of infections during chemotherapy treatment.

Enhanced Cancer Treatment Efficacy:

Studies suggest that turkey tail mushroom extracts have anti-tumor properties. They may work synergistically with chemotherapy drugs to enhance their effectiveness against cancer cells. Research has shown that the polysaccharides in turkey tail can inhibit tumor growth, induce apoptosis (programmed cell death), and inhibit metastasis in various cancer types.

Reduction of Chemotherapy Side Effects:

Chemotherapy commonly causes side effects such as nausea, vomiting, fatigue, and immune suppression. Turkey tail mushroom's immunomodulatory and antioxidant properties may help alleviate some of these side effects. By supporting immune function and reducing oxidative stress, it could potentially enhance overall well-being and quality of life for cancer patients undergoing chemotherapy.

Clinical Studies and Evidence:

While many studies have been conducted in vitro (in the lab) and in animal models, clinical trials in humans are ongoing to validate the efficacy and safety of turkey tail mushroom alongside chemotherapy. Some clinical trials have shown promising results, particularly in terms of immune system enhancement and tolerability of chemotherapy.

Safety and Considerations:

Turkey tail mushroom is considered safe for consumption when taken as a supplement or in the form of extracts. However, like any supplement, quality, dosage, and purity are crucial factors. It's essential for patients to consult with their healthcare providers before using turkey tail mushroom alongside chemotherapy to ensure compatibility with their treatment plan and to monitor for any potential interactions or adverse effects.

Integrative Approach:

Integrating complementary therapies like turkey tail mushroom with conventional cancer treatments such as chemotherapy is part of the field of integrative oncology. This approach aims to optimize treatment outcomes while improving quality of life for cancer patients.

Conclusion

While turkey tail mushroom shows promise as a supportive therapy alongside chemotherapy, further research, particularly large-scale clinical trials, is needed to establish its efficacy, safety, and optimal usage in cancer treatment protocols. Consulting healthcare professionals and incorporating evidence-based integrative approaches remain crucial for personalized cancer care.

Testimonies of turkey tail mushroom

Judy's Story

Testimony: Judy was diagnosed with stage 4 breast cancer and given a prognosis of just a few months. After learning about the benefits of medicinal mushrooms, she incorporated turkey tail supplements daily into her treatment. She also continued with her chemotherapy. Judy reported feeling stronger, more energetic, and ultimately found that her tumors had shrunk significantly. She attributes much of her improved well-being and potential remission to the use of turkey tail mushrooms.

Paul Stamets' Mother

Testimony: Dr. Paul Stamets, a renowned mycologist, shared the story of his mother, who had stage 4 breast cancer. She started taking high doses of turkey tail mushroom supplements after her diagnosis. Over time, her tumors showed significant reduction, and she surpassed the expected survival timeframe. Dr. Stamets has since advocated for the use of turkey tail mushrooms in cancer treatment, using his mother's experience as an example.

Ken S.

Testimony: Ken, a colorectal cancer patient, shared on a cancer support forum how he started using turkey tail mushroom supplements along with chemotherapy. He noticed fewer side effects from his treatment and an improvement in his overall energy. While he continued with his conventional treatment, he felt that the turkey tail helped keep his immune system strong and contributed to an improved quality of life.

Linda B.

Testimony: Linda, who had recurrent ovarian cancer, began taking turkey tail mushrooms after her second round of treatment. She found that the mushroom supplement supported her immune system, which allowed her to maintain better health throughout her chemotherapy sessions. Linda was pleased with the decrease in her usual side effects and said she felt "like herself" more often than she did during her initial treatment without turkey tail.

James W.

Testimony: James, diagnosed with lung cancer, integrated turkey tail mushrooms into his holistic treatment plan. He reported an unexpected stabilization of his tumor size, which he initially attributed to diet and lifestyle changes. However, he later learned more about turkey tail's immune-boosting properties and credited his stable condition partly to the mushrooms.

Hyperbaric Oxygen Therapy

HBOT involves breathing pure oxygen in a pressurized room or chamber. It's primarily used for conditions like chronic wounds, decompression sickness, and certain infections. However, its application in cancer treatment is an area of ongoing research and interest.

How HBOT Works

Increased Oxygen Delivery: The high pressure increases the amount of oxygen dissolved in the blood plasma, which can enhance oxygen delivery to tissues.

Anti-Inflammatory Effects: HBOT may reduce inflammation and promote wound healing.

Neovascularization: It can stimulate the growth of new blood vessels, which might help in healing tissues damaged by radiation therapy.

Potential Benefits of HBOT in Cancer Treatment

Enhanced Radiation Therapy:

Mechanism: HBOT increases the amount of oxygen in the blood and tissues, which can enhance the effectiveness of radiation therapy. Oxygen is known to improve the efficacy of radiation by making cancer cells more susceptible to damage.

Research Findings: Some studies have shown that HBOT can improve the outcomes of radiation therapy by enhancing tumor oxygenation and potentially increasing the therapeutic ratio.

Reduction of Radiation-Induced Tissue Damage:

Mechanism: By promoting healing and reducing inflammation, HBOT may help mitigate radiation-induced damage to surrounding healthy tissues.

Research Findings: Clinical trials have indicated that HBOT can reduce the severity of radiation-induced side effects such as fibrosis, ulcers, and tissue necrosis.

Improved Wound Healing:

Mechanism: The therapy's ability to stimulate neovascularization (the formation of new blood vessels) can accelerate wound healing, which may be beneficial for patients with surgical wounds or radiation-induced injuries.

Research Findings: Evidence suggests that HBOT can enhance the healing of chronic wounds and tissue damage resulting from cancer treatment.

Symptom Management:

Mechanism: HBOT may alleviate symptoms like pain and fatigue by improving overall tissue oxygenation and reducing inflammation.

Research Findings: Some studies have reported improvements in quality-of-life measures and symptom management among patients undergoing HBOT.

Areas of Concern and Limitations

Mixed Evidence on Efficacy:

Concern: The research on HBOT's effectiveness in cancer treatment is not uniformly positive. Some studies have found minimal or no benefit.

Current State: The evidence is still evolving, with some trials showing promising results while others suggest limited impact.

Potential for Tumor Growth Stimulation:

Concern: There is a theoretical risk that increased oxygenation could potentially stimulate the growth of certain tumors, particularly those that are highly vascularized.

Current State: This concern is based on the premise that oxygen could support tumor metabolism and growth, though more research is needed to clarify this risk.

Lack of Standardized Protocols:

Concern: The optimal parameters for HBOT, such as pressure levels, duration, and frequency, are not well established for cancer patients.

Current State: Variability in treatment protocols and a lack of consensus on best practices can lead to inconsistent outcomes and challenges in clinical application.

Cost and Accessibility:

Concern: HBOT can be expensive and may not be covered by all insurance plans, limiting its accessibility for some patients.

Current State: The cost of HBOT and its availability may pose barriers to its widespread use in cancer care.

Conclusion

HBOT holds potential benefits for cancer patients, particularly in enhancing radiation therapy effectiveness, reducing side effects, and improving wound healing. However, concerns about mixed research results, potential tumor growth stimulation, and lack of standardized protocols highlight the need for further investigation. Ongoing research will be crucial in determining the precise role of HBOT in cancer treatment and ensuring its safe and effective application.

Testimonies of HBOT

Susan R.:

"After my radiation therapy for breast cancer, I developed severe skin damage. My doctor recommended HBOT, and I was amazed at how quickly my skin healed. The pain diminished, and I felt a renewed sense of hope during my recovery."

James L.:

"Following my treatment for prostate cancer, I struggled with fatigue and recovery. HBOT helped me regain my energy and improved my overall health. I believe it played a significant role in my healing process."

Karen M.:

"I was diagnosed with cervical cancer and underwent extensive treatment. After my surgery, I started HBOT to aid in healing. The sessions made a noticeable difference in my recovery, and I felt better physically and mentally."

Robert T.:

"After battling head and neck cancer, I experienced chronic pain and tissue damage from radiation. My oncologist suggested HBOT, and I noticed a marked improvement in my healing. It felt like a breath of fresh air during a tough time."

Emily J.:

"Dealing with the aftereffects of lung cancer treatment was daunting. I added HBOT to my regimen, and it helped with my breathing and energy levels. I'm grateful for the positive impact it had on my life."

Natural Vitamins

While undergoing chemotherapy, it is crucial to prioritize those that can support overall health, manage side effects, and complement conventional treatment without interfering with its efficacy. Here are some commonly recommended natural vitamins and supplements:

Vitamin D

Many cancer patients are deficient in vitamin D, which plays a crucial role in immune function and bone health. Chemotherapy can further deplete vitamin D levels. Supplementing vitamin D under healthcare provider guidance can help maintain optimal levels.

Omega-3 Fatty Acids

Found in fish oil supplements, omega-3 fatty acids have anti-inflammatory properties and may help reduce inflammation caused by chemotherapy. They also support cardiovascular health.

Probiotics

Chemotherapy can disrupt gut flora, leading to digestive issues. Probiotics help maintain gut health and may alleviate symptoms like diarrhea and nausea.

B Vitamins

Chemotherapy can sometimes lead to deficiencies in B vitamins such as B6, B12, and folate. These vitamins are essential for energy production, nerve function, and DNA synthesis.

Antioxidants

Certain antioxidants like vitamin C, vitamin E, and selenium can help combat oxidative stress caused by chemotherapy. However, their use alongside treatment should be monitored to avoid interference with chemotherapy's mechanisms.

Glutamine

This amino acid supports the digestive tract lining and may help reduce mucositis (inflammation and ulcers in the mouth and digestive tract) caused by chemotherapy.

Curcumin

Found in turmeric, curcumin has anti-inflammatory and antioxidant properties. It may help alleviate inflammation and support overall health during chemotherapy.

Melatonin

Some studies suggest melatonin may help improve sleep quality, which can be disrupted during chemotherapy treatment. Always consult with your healthcare provider before starting any new supplements, as they can advise on appropriate dosages, potential interactions with chemotherapy drugs, and monitor your health throughout treatment. Individual needs vary, and personalized recommendations based on your specific health status and treatment regimen are essential for safety and efficacy.

Natural Home Remedies

Combining chemotherapy with natural home remedies can help manage side effects and improve overall well-being. However, it is crucial to consult with a healthcare provider before starting any new remedies to avoid potential interactions with cancer treatments.

Ginger

Ginger is widely known for its anti-nausea properties, which can be particularly helpful for chemotherapy-induced nausea and vomiting. It can be consumed as tea, fresh ginger, or ginger supplements.

Turmeric

Turmeric contains curcumin, which has anti-inflammatory and antioxidant properties. It can help reduce inflammation and support the immune system. Turmeric can be added to food or taken as a supplement.

Peppermint

Peppermint can help alleviate nausea and digestive issues. Peppermint tea or peppermint oil capsules are common ways to consume it. It also has a calming effect, which can reduce anxiety.

Aloe Vera

Aloe vera can soothe the skin and help with mouth sores, a common side effect of chemotherapy. Drinking aloe vera juice can also aid in digestive health.

Probiotics

Choosing the best probiotic while undergoing chemotherapy can help manage side effects like diarrhea, nausea, and general gut health. Here are some top recommendations based on their strain composition, quality, and compatibility with chemotherapy:

VSL#3

Strains: Contains a mix of 8 different probiotic strains, including Lactobacillus, Bifidobacterium, and Streptococcus thermophilus.

Benefits: Known for its high potency and effectiveness in managing gastrointestinal issues, which can be particularly beneficial during chemotherapy.

Research: Has been studied for its effects in managing inflammatory bowel diseases and other gut-related conditions.

Florastor

Strains: Contains Saccharomyces boulardii, a beneficial yeast.

Benefits: Effective in preventing antibiotic-associated diarrhea and may help with maintaining gut flora during chemotherapy.

Research: Several studies support its use in managing diarrhea and improving gut health.

Culturelle Digestive Health

Strains: Contains Lactobacillus rhamnosus GG.

Benefits: Known for its robust research backing and effectiveness in improving overall gut health and reducing diarrhea.

Research: Extensively studied and shown to be effective in various gastrointestinal conditions.

Align Probiotic

Strains: Contains Bifidobacterium longum 35624.

Benefits: Particularly effective in managing irritable bowel syndrome (IBS) and maintaining gut health.

Research: Well-researched and shown to support digestive health and regularity.

Renew Life Ultimate Flora Probiotic

Strains: Contains a blend of multiple strains, including Lactobacillus and Bifidobacterium.

Benefits: High CFU count, and variety of strains can help maintain a balanced gut flora.

Research: Known for its high quality and effectiveness in promoting digestive health.

Consult Your Healthcare Provider

Personalized Advice: Your oncologist or healthcare provider can recommend specific probiotics based on your individual health needs and treatment plan.

Green Tea

Green tea is rich in antioxidants and has anti-inflammatory properties. Drinking green tea can support the immune system and provide a gentle energy boost.

Echinacea

Echinacea is known for boosting the immune system. It can be taken as a tea or supplement to help support immune health during chemotherapy.

Omega-3 Fatty Acids

Fish Oil Supplements

Look for high-quality fish oil supplements, particularly those derived from fatty fishlike salmon, mackerel, sardines, and anchovies. These are rich in EPA (eicosapentaenoic acid) and DHA (docosahexaenoic acid).

Purity: opt for molecularly distilled fish oils, which have impurities and heavy metals removed.

Packaging: Choose supplements that come in dark or opaque bottles to protect against light exposure, which can cause oxidation.

Krill Oil

Benefits: Krill oil is rich in EPA and DHA, bound to phospholipids, which can enhance absorption. It also contains astaxanthin, a powerful antioxidant that helps prevent oxidation.

Stability: Krill oil is more stable than fish oil due to its natural antioxidant content, reducing the risk of oxidation.

Algal Oil

Vegan Option: Algal oil is derived from algae and is a good source of DHA, making it suitable for vegetarians and vegans.

Sustainability: It is considered a sustainable source of omega-3s and typically has a lower risk of contamination compared to fish oil.

Least Oxidation Risk

Packaging and Storage

Dark Bottles: Omega-3 supplements should be stored in dark, airtight containers to protect them from light and air, both of which can accelerate oxidation.

Refrigeration: Storing omega-3 supplements in the refrigerator can slow down the oxidation process and extend shelf life.

Antioxidant Additives

Vitamin E: Many high-quality omega-3 supplements include vitamin E (tocopherol) as an antioxidant to prevent oxidation.

Astaxanthin: In krill oil, astaxanthin acts as a natural antioxidant, providing extra protection against oxidation.

Choose Reputable Brands

Third-Party Testing: Select products from reputable brands that offer third-party testing for purity and oxidation levels. Look for certifications from organizations like IFOS (International Fish Oil Standards) or GOED (Global Organization for EPA and DHA Omega-3s).

Natural Sources

Fatty Fish: Consuming fresh, fatty fish like salmon, mackerel, and sardines are an excellent way to obtain omega-3s with minimal oxidation risk, provided the fish is fresh and properly stored.

Flaxseeds and Chia Seeds: While plant-based sources like flaxseeds and chia seeds provide ALA (alpha-linolenic acid), which the body can partially convert to EPA and DHA, they are a suitable alternative for those who prefer plant-based options.

Vitamin D

Vitamin D3 (Cholecalciferol)

Absorption: Vitamin D3 is more effective at raising and supporting vitamin D levels in the blood compared to D2 (ergocalciferol).

Sources: D3 can be obtained from supplements, fatty fish, liver, egg yolks, and fortified foods.

Supplement Form: Look for high-quality vitamin D3 supplements. Many healthcare professionals recommend a dosage tailored to your individual needs, which might be found through blood tests.

Vitamin K

Vitamin K2 (Menaquinone)

Types of K2: There are several forms of K2, but MK-7 and MK-4 are the most common and studied.

MK-7: Long half-life, meaning it stays in the blood longer. Found in fermented foods like natto.

MK-4: Shorter half-life but beneficial for bone and cardiovascular health. Found in animal products and available as supplements.

Absorption and Effectiveness: K2 is generally considered more effective than K1 (phylloquinone) in supporting bone and cardiovascular health.

Synergistic Effect: Vitamins D3 and K2 work synergistically. D3 aids calcium absorption, while K2 helps direct calcium to the bones, preventing arterial calcification.

Combined Supplements: Some supplements contain both D3 and K2, offering a convenient way to ensure you're getting both vitamins in the right amounts.

Hydration

Using Celtic salt or Himalayan salt before hydrating can provide additional benefits by replenishing electrolytes and minerals, which are essential for maintaining fluid balance and overall health, especially during chemotherapy.

Benefits of Celtic Salt and Himalayan Salt for Hydration

Mineral Content

Celtic Salt: Contains over 80 trace minerals, including magnesium, potassium, and calcium, which help in maintaining electrolyte balance and proper hydration.

Himalayan Salt: Rich in minerals like iron, magnesium, calcium, and potassium. It also contains around 84 trace minerals that support various bodily functions.

Electrolyte Balance

Hydration: Adding a small amount of these salts to your water can enhance hydration by providing essential electrolytes that help the body absorb and retain fluids more effectively.

Muscle Function: The minerals in these salts support muscle function and can help reduce cramps, which may be beneficial during chemotherapy when muscle weakness and cramps can be an issue.

How to Use Celtic Salt or Himalayan Salt

Salt Sole Solution

Preparation: Create a salt sole by dissolving Himalayan or Celtic salt in water until it becomes saturated (i.e., the salt no longer dissolves).
Typically, this involves adding a few tablespoons of salt to a glass jar of water and allowing it to sit for 24 hours.

Usage: Add a teaspoon of the sole solution to a glass of water in the morning. This can help kickstart your hydration and replenish electrolytes.

Adding to Water

Direct Addition: Add a pinch of Himalayan or Celtic salt directly to your water bottle. This method is quick and can be done throughout the day to maintain electrolyte levels.

Flavor Enhancement: For added flavor and benefits, combine it with lemon or lime juice, which provides additional vitamins and makes the water more palatable.

Balanced Diet

Maintaining a balanced diet rich in fruits, vegetables, lean proteins, and whole grains provides essential nutrients that support overall health and recovery during chemotherapy.

Key Considerations

Consult with your doctor: Always discuss any new supplements or dietary changes with your healthcare provider to ensure they are safe and will not interfere with your treatment.

Monitor for interactions: Some natural remedies may interact with chemotherapy drugs, so professional guidance is crucial.

Stay informed: Keep up with reliable sources of information and support groups for cancer patients to share experiences and recommendations.

Combining these natural remedies with your chemotherapy regimen can help manage side effects and improve quality of life.

Detoxification and Cleansing Methods

Detoxification involves eliminating toxins from the body to improve health and well-being. Here are some effective detoxification methods:

Hydration

Importance: Water flushes out toxins from the body through urine and sweat.

How to Use: Aim for at least 8-10 glasses of water daily. Adding lemon to water can enhance detoxification due to its antioxidant properties.

Dietary Changes

Whole Foods: Emphasize fresh fruits, vegetables, lean proteins, and whole grains.

Fiber-Rich Foods: Fiber aids digestion and helps remove toxins from the digestive tract. Include foods like oats, flaxseeds, and leafy greens.

Avoid Processed Foods: Limit intake of processed foods, refined sugars, and unhealthy fats.

Herbal Teas

Dandelion Root Tea: Supports liver function and acts as a diuretic, helping to eliminate toxins through urine.

Green Tea: Rich in antioxidants, green tea can enhance liver function and detoxification processes.

Exercise

Benefits: Physical activity promotes circulation and sweating, which helps expel toxins through the skin.

Recommendations: Aim for at least 30 minutes of moderate exercise daily, such as walking, jogging, or yoga.

Intermittent Fasting

How it Works: Intermittent fasting involves cycles of eating and fasting. This can give the digestive system a break and allow the body to focus on repair and detoxification.

Common methods include the 16/8 method (16 hours fasting, 8 hours eating).

Sauna Therapy

Benefits: Regular sauna use promotes sweating, which helps eliminate toxins through the skin.
Usage: Start with shorter sessions and gradually increase time as tolerated.

Importance of Liver Health

The liver is a key organ in detoxification, responsible for filtering blood and metabolizing toxins. Supporting liver health is crucial for effective detoxification.

Detoxifying Foods for Liver Health

Cruciferous Vegetables

Examples: Broccoli, Brussels sprouts, cabbage.
Benefits: High in sulfur compounds and antioxidants, they support liver enzyme production and detoxification pathways.

Garlic

Benefits: Contains allicin and selenium, which help cleanse the liver and activate liver enzymes that flush out toxins.

Turmeric

Benefits: Curcumin, the active ingredient, has anti-inflammatory and antioxidant properties that support liver function and detoxification.

Citrus Fruits

Examples: Lemons, oranges, grapefruits.
Benefits: High in vitamin C and antioxidants, citrus fruits enhance liver detoxification and support the immune system.

Green Leafy Vegetables

Examples: Spinach, kale, arugula.
Benefits: Rich in chlorophyll, they help detoxify the liver by neutralizing heavy metals, chemicals, and pesticides.

Beets and Carrots

Benefits: High in beta-carotene and plant-flavonoids, which can stimulate and improve overall liver function.

Avocados

Benefits: Rich in healthy fats and antioxidants, avocados help the body produce glutathione, a compound essential for liver detoxification.

Holistic Approach to Cancer Prevention

Stress management is a crucial aspect of holistic cancer prevention, as chronic stress has been linked to inflammation, weakened immune function, and potentially increased cancer risk.

Here are some holistic approaches to stress management that can contribute to cancer prevention:

Mindfulness Meditation:

Mindfulness practices, such as meditation and deep breathing exercises, can help reduce stress levels. They promote relaxation and improve resilience to stressors.

Exercise:

Regular physical activity is not only beneficial for physical health but also for mental well-being. Exercise releases endorphins, which are natural mood lifters, and helps to reduce stress hormones like cortisol.

Nature and Outdoor Activities:

Spending time in nature or engaging in outdoor activities can lower stress levels and promote a sense of calm. Even a short walk in a park can have positive effects on mental health.

Social Support:

Strong social connections and relationships provide emotional support during stressful times. Talking with friends, family, or joining support groups can help alleviate stress.

Healthy Lifestyle:

Adopting a healthy lifestyle, including a balanced diet, regular sleep patterns, and avoiding substances like alcohol and tobacco, can all contribute to better stress management and overall well-being.

Time Management:

Effective time management can reduce feelings of being overwhelmed and stressed. Prioritizing tasks, setting realistic goals, and learning to say no when necessary are important skills.

Cognitive Behavioral Therapy (CBT):

CBT techniques can help individuals identify and change negative thought patterns and behaviors that contribute to stress.

Art and Creative Activities:

Engaging in creative activities such as painting, writing, or music can provide a therapeutic outlet for stress and emotions.

Relaxation Techniques:

Techniques such as progressive muscle relaxation, guided imagery, and aromatherapy can promote relaxation and reduce stress.

It is important to remember that everyone responds to stress differently, so finding the right combination of stress management techniques that work for you is key. By incorporating these holistic approaches into your daily life, you can effectively manage stress levels and potentially reduce your risk of cancer by supporting overall health and well-being.

A Prayer for Peace and Strength

Heavenly Father,

In this time of overwhelming challenge, I come before You seeking Your comfort and peace. The journey through cancer is fraught with fear, uncertainty, and physical suffering, and I ask for Your grace to ease my burden.

Grant me the strength to face each day with courage and resilience. Help me to find moments of calm amidst the storm, and to feel Your presence guiding me through this difficult path. May Your peace, which surpasses all understanding, guard my heart and mind, soothing the waves of anxiety that wash over me.

Lord, I pray for patience as I navigate the treatments and their side effects. Surround me with Your healing light, and let it fill my body, mind, and spirit with hope and positivity. I trust in Your divine plan, even when the road ahead seems uncertain. Bless my loved ones who support me, giving them strength and understanding. May they be a source of comfort and encouragement, as I am to them. Guide the hands and minds of the medical professionals caring for me, granting them wisdom and compassion.

Help me to find solace in the small blessings each day brings, and to remain grateful for the love and support that surrounds me. Teach me to release my worries into Your capable hands, and to rest in the knowledge that I am never alone.

In Your name, I find peace. In Your love, I find healing. In Your strength, I find the courage to face tomorrow.

Amen.

A Prayer for Miracle Healing

Heavenly Father,

I come before You with a heart full of hope and faith, seeking Your miraculous touch. You are the God of wonders, the healer of the sick, and the source of all life. In my time of need, I turn to You, believing in Your power to heal and restore.

Lord, I ask for Your divine intervention in my body, mind, and spirit. Touch me with Your healing hands and remove every trace of illness and pain. Breathe new life into my cells, tissues, and organs, and bring complete and total healing to every part of my being.

I trust in Your mercy and grace, knowing that nothing is impossible for You. Strengthen my faith as I wait for Your healing and grant me the patience to endure the trials I face. Surround me with Your peace, and let Your presence be a constant source of comfort and reassurance.

Lord, I also lift up to You the doctors, nurses, and caregivers who are involved in my care. Bless them with wisdom, compassion, and the skills they need to bring about the best possible outcomes. Guide their hands and hearts as they work to restore my health.

Help me to find strength in my faith and to lean on You in moments of doubt and fear. Remind me of Your promises and Your love, which never fails. Fill me with the light of Your healing power, and let it radiate through me, bringing hope and encouragement to those around me.

I thank You, Lord, for the healing that is already taking place within me. I believe in Your miraculous power and trust that You are working in my life, even when I cannot see it. May Your will be done, and may Your name be glorified through my healing.

In Jesus' name, I pray,

Amen.

Fasting

There is emerging research suggesting that fasting may have a potential relationship with cancer treatment, primarily through mechanisms that affect cancer cell metabolism and enhance the effectiveness of conventional treatments.

Here are some key points on the relationship between fasting and cancer:

Mechanisms

Reduced Glucose Availability:

> Cancer cells typically have a high demand for glucose due to their rapid growth and reliance on glycolysis (Warburg effect). Fasting reduces blood glucose levels, potentially starving cancer cells of their primary energy source.

Ketosis:

> is a metabolic state in which the body primarily uses fat for fuel instead of carbohydrates. This occurs when carbohydrate intake is significantly reduced, leading the liver to produce ketones from fatty acids. Some research suggests that ketosis may have potential benefits in the context of cancer treatment, although the topic is still under investigation.

Here are a few ways ketosis might influence cancer:

Altered Energy Metabolism:

> Cancer cells often rely on glucose for energy. By reducing carbohydrate intake and promoting ketosis, the availability of glucose can be limited, potentially slowing the growth of certain tumors.

Ketones as Fuel:

Some studies suggest that healthy cells can adapt to using ketones for energy, while cancer cells may struggle with this shift, which could impair their growth and proliferation.

Reduced Insulin Levels:

A ketogenic diet can lower insulin levels, which may help reduce the growth signals that some cancers respond to.
Improved Oxidative Stress:
Ketones can produce less reactive oxygen species compared to glucose metabolism, potentially leading to a less favorable environment for cancer cells.

Potential Synergistic Effects with Treatments:

Some research shows that a ketogenic diet may enhance the effectiveness of certain cancer treatments, such as chemotherapy and radiation.

Reduced Insulin and IGF-1 Levels:

Fasting lowers levels of insulin and insulin-like growth factor 1 (IGF-1), both of which can promote cancer cell proliferation. Reduced levels of these hormones may slow down cancer growth.

Autophagy:

Fasting induces autophagy, a cellular process that cleans up damaged cells and proteins. This can lead to the destruction of cancer cells and improve the overall health of cells.

Enhanced Chemotherapy and Radiation Sensitivity:

Some studies suggest that fasting can make cancer cells more sensitive to chemotherapy and radiation, potentially enhancing the effectiveness of these treatments while protecting normal cells from their toxic effects.

Research and Evidence

Animal Studies:

Numerous animal studies have shown that fasting can slow tumor growth and improve the effectiveness of cancer treatments. For example, fasting has been shown to increase the susceptibility of cancer cells to chemotherapy.

Human Studies:

Clinical trials in humans are still limited, but early studies show promising results. Some small studies have shown that fasting before and during chemotherapy can reduce side effects and improve treatment outcomes.
A study published in "Science Translational Medicine" (2012) found that short-term fasting protected mice against high-dose chemotherapy while enhancing its effectiveness against cancer.

Another study in "Cell Metabolism" (2016) showed that fasting-mimicking diets (low-calorie, low-protein diets that mimic the effects of fasting) can reduce the risk factors and biomarkers associated with aging and diseases, including cancer.

Practical Considerations

Medical Supervision:

Fasting, especially prolonged fasting, should be done under medical supervision, particularly for cancer patients. Nutritional status, overall health, and treatment plans need to be carefully managed.

Individual Variability:

Responses to fasting can vary significantly among individuals. Factors such as cancer type, stage, overall health, and concurrent treatments need to be.

Types of Fasting

Intermittent Fasting

Definition: Alternating periods of eating and fasting. Common methods include the 16/8 method (fast for 16 hours and eat during an 8-hour window) and the 5:2 method (eating normally for 5 days and reducing calorie intake for 2 non-consecutive days).

Purpose: May help reduce inflammation, improve metabolism, and enhance cellular repair processes.

Water Fasting

Definition: Consuming only water for a set period, usually 24-72 hours.

Purpose: Can promote autophagy (cellular cleanup) and potentially improve the effectiveness of cancer treatments. Should be medically supervised.

Juice Fasting

Definition: Consuming only fruit and vegetable juices for nutrition over time.

Purpose: Provides vitamins and antioxidants while giving the digestive system a break. Popular for detoxification and to consume concentrated nutrients.

Fermented Enzymes Fasting

These are enzymes derived from the fermentation of foods. Fermentation is a process where microorganisms like bacteria or yeast break down food substances. Common fermented foods include kimchi, sauerkraut, miso, and kombucha. Enzymes produced during fermentation can aid in digestion and support overall health.

The Concept of Fermented Enzymes and Fasting

Digestive Support: Fermented enzymes are thought to enhance digestion and nutrient absorption, potentially making the fasting process easier by reducing digestive stress.

Detoxification: Some proponents believe that fermented enzymes can aid in detoxification, helping to clear out toxins from the body. This is thought to complement the detoxifying effects of fasting.

Immune Support: Fermented foods are often rich in probiotics, which can support gut health and, by extension, boost the immune system. A strong immune system is crucial in cancer treatment.

Regimens

Baking Soda and Celtic Saltwater Regimen

Morning: Drink a glass of water with 1/4 teaspoon of baking soda and a pinch of Celtic salt.

Throughout the Day: Continue to drink plain water and add baking soda water (up to 2 times more) if needed.

Irish Sea Moss Regimen

Preparation: Soak 1/4 cup of Irish sea moss in water overnight. Blend into a gel.

Morning: Drink a glass of water mixed with 1-2 tablespoons of Irish sea moss gel.

Throughout the Day: Drink water and consume the Irish sea moss gel as needed, up to 1/2 cup total per day.

Water and Juice Fasting Regimen

Morning: Start with a glass of water.

Mid-Morning: Drink a glass of fresh vegetable juice (e.g., carrot, celery, spinach).

Lunchtime: Another glass of water, followed by fruit juice (e.g., apple, beet, lemon).

Afternoon: Alternate between water and vegetable/fruit juices every few hours.

Evening: Finish with a glass of water and a light juice, such as cucumber or watermelon.

Fermented Enzymes and Fasting

Preparation: Choose a fasting method (e.g., water fasting or juice fasting] and incorporate fermented enzyme supplements as directed.

During Fasting: Take fermented enzyme supplements according to the recommended dosage. These can be in the form of capsules, powders, or liquid extracts.

Hydration: Drink plenty of water throughout the fasting period.

Post-Fasting: Gradually reintroduce foods with the support of fermented enzymes to aid digestion and absorption.

Testimonies of fasting

Vernon Johnston

Experience: "I began a regimen of fasting to starve the cancer cells of sugar, which they thrive on. I combined this with an alkaline diet and regular baking soda with molasses to keep my body's pH in a cancer-fighting state. Over time, my PSA levels dropped, and follow-up scans showed significant improvements. My doctors were skeptical, but the results were clear. While I cannot say fasting alone cured my cancer, I believe it played a

John D.

Experience: "After my surgery, I was determined to do everything in my power to prevent the cancer from coming back. I read about the potential benefits of fasting and decided to give it a try. I started with intermittent fasting and gradually worked up to longer fasts of 3-5 days. I noticed that my energy levels improved, and my digestive system felt more balanced. Most importantly, my follow-up scans have remained clear, and my oncologist has been impressed with my overall health. Fasting, combined with a healthy diet and lifestyle changes, has been an integral part of my cancer-free journey."

Patricia K.

Experience: "When I was diagnosed with breast cancer, I underwent surgery and chemotherapy. Alongside these treatments, I started practicing intermittent fasting and occasionally did longer fasts. I read that fasting could help improve the effectiveness of chemotherapy and protect normal cells from its toxic effects. During my fasting periods, I felt less nauseous and had more energy. My oncologist noted that I handled the chemotherapy better than most patients. While I followed all medical advice, I believe that fasting helped me manage the side effects and possibly contributed to my remission."

Mark Simon

Experience: "Diagnosed with an aggressive form of lymphoma, I decided to take a comprehensive approach to my treatment. This included a strict ketogenic diet, regular fasting, and conventional therapies like chemotherapy. During fasting periods, I felt my body was in a healing state. I experienced clearer thinking and a sense of empowerment over my health. Over time, my tumor markers decreased, and my scans showed significant regression. I attribute my recovery to a combination of medical treatments and the fasting protocol I adhered to."

Jane McLelland

Experience: "My battle with stage IV cancer was daunting, but I chose to fight it with every possible tool. Fasting became a key part of my strategy, along with a low-carbohydrate diet and supplements. Fasting helped me feel more in control and seemed to enhance the effectiveness of my other treatments. My scans began to show improvement, and my doctors were amazed at my progress. I believe that fasting played a vital role in my recovery, giving my body the edge, it needed to combat the cancer."

Prayer

For cancer patients seeking solace and encouragement in biblical scripture, here are several passages that are often comforting and uplifting:

Psalm 23:4:

> "Even though I walk through the darkest valley, I will fear no evil, for you are with me; your rod and your staff, they comfort me."

Isaiah 41:10:

> "So do not fear, for I am with you; do not be dismayed, for I am your God. I will strengthen you and help you; I will uphold you with my righteous right hand."

Philippians 4:6-7:

> "Do not be anxious about anything, but in every situation, by prayer and petition, with thanksgiving, present your requests to God. And the peace of God, which transcends all understanding, will guard your hearts and your minds in Christ Jesus."

James 5:14-15:

> "Is anyone among you sick? Let them call the elders of the church to pray over them and anoint them with oil in the name of the Lord. And the prayer offered in faith will make the sick person well; the Lord will raise them up. If they have sinned, they will be forgiven."

2 Corinthians 4:16-18:

> "Therefore, we do not lose heart. Though outwardly we are wasting away, yet inwardly we are being renewed day by day. For our light and momentary troubles are achieving for us an eternal glory that far outweighs them all. So, we fix our

> eyes not on what is seen, but on what is unseen, since what is seen is temporary, but what is unseen is eternal."

Romans 8:38-39:

> "For I am convinced that neither death nor life, neither angels nor demons, neither the present nor the future, nor any powers, neither height nor depth, nor anything else in all creation, will be able to separate us from the love of God that is in Christ Jesus our Lord."

These scriptures emphasize themes of strength, faith, peace, and the assurance of God's presence and love during difficult times. They can provide comfort and a sense of hope to those facing the challenges of cancer.

Testimonies of Prayer

Sarah's Story:

> *Testimony:* "I was diagnosed with aggressive stage 4 breast cancer and given a grim prognosis. Devastated, I turned to prayer and sought the support of my church community. Over months of intense prayer and unwavering faith, my scans began to show unexpected improvements. Eventually, doctors were amazed to find no evidence of cancer remaining. I attribute my healing to the power of prayer and God's grace."

John's Journey:

> *Testimony:* "Facing a terminal diagnosis of stage 4 lung cancer, I leaned heavily on prayer and the support of my family and church. Despite grim medical predictions, I experienced a gradual improvement in my health over time. Scans began to show shrinking tumors and eventually no signs of cancer at all. My doctors were astounded and attributed my recovery to a

combination of treatments and the spiritual strength I gained through prayer."

Mary's Miracle:

Testimony: "When I was diagnosed with stage 4 pancreatic cancer, I knew the odds were against me. With the encouragement of my faith community, I prayed fervently for healing. Despite the aggressive nature of my cancer, subsequent tests began to show regression of tumors until they completely disappeared. My medical team was amazed and acknowledged the remarkable turnaround as something beyond medical explanation."

Mandi McLeod:

Mandi was diagnosed with stage 4 cancer and shares her journey of faith and healing through her blog and social media. While her story may not be as widely known as the others, it resonates with many who have faced similar battles.

Cancer Treatment Centers that don't use Chemotherapy

Hippocrates Health Institute (West Palm Beach, Florida, USA):
Known for its holistic approach to health and wellness, including cancer treatment.
Emphasizes raw vegan diets, juicing, detoxification, and mind-body therapies.

Gerson Institute (San Diego, California, USA):
Follows the Gerson Therapy, which includes a strict organic plant-based diet, juicing, detoxification, and supplements.
Focuses on boosting the body's immune system and eliminating toxins.

An Oasis of Healing (Mesa, Arizona, USA):
Integrative oncology clinic offering treatments that combine conventional and alternative therapies.
Emphasizes nutrition, detoxification, immune support, and mind-body approaches.
Issels® Integrative Immuno-Oncology (Santa Barbara, California, USA):
Offers integrative cancer treatments that include immunotherapy, nutrition, detoxification, and lifestyle changes.
Focuses on enhancing the body's immune response to fight cancer naturally.

Hope4Cancer Treatment Centers (Multiple locations including Cancun, Mexico):
It provides integrative cancer therapies that incorporate non-toxic treatments such as hyperthermia, detoxification, and immune support.
Focuses on addressing the underlying causes of cancer and supporting overall health.
Oasis of Hope Hospital (Tijuana, Mexico):
Offers alternative cancer treatments including nutritional therapies, immune support, and lifestyle changes.

Focuses on holistic healing and personalized treatment plans.

The Budwig Center (Malaga, Spain):
Follows the Budwig Protocol, which includes a specific diet (based on flaxseed oil and cottage cheese), detoxification, and supplementation. Emphasizes cellular health and strengthening the immune system. It is important to approach any alternative cancer treatment center with caution and do thorough research. Look for centers that prioritize safety, evidence-based practices, and transparency about their success rates and patient outcomes. Always consult with healthcare professionals and consider seeking multiple opinions before making decisions about cancer treatment.

Summary of References

Simopoulos, A. P. (2002) - This article discusses the critical balance between omega-6 and omega-3 fatty acids in the diet, highlighting its significance in human health and potential implications for various diseases, including cancer.

Lands, W. E. (2015) - This historical review examines the impact of omega-3 and omega-6 nutrients on health, tracing their roles in disease prevention and promoting overall wellness, particularly in relation to heart health.

Paniangvait et al. (1995) - The study investigates cholesterol oxides in animal-derived foods, providing insights into their formation and potential health implications, including links to cancer risk.

Shahidi, F., & Zhong, Y. (2010) - This review focuses on lipid oxidation and methods to improve oxidative stability, emphasizing the importance of preventing oxidative damage in foods, which is relevant to cancer prevention strategies.

Mozaffarian et al. (2006) - The research discusses the adverse effects of trans fatty acids on cardiovascular health, linking them to increased risk of heart disease and other metabolic disorders.

Micha, R., & Mozaffarian, D. (2009) - This article reviews the effects of trans fatty acids on metabolic syndrome, heart disease, and diabetes, highlighting the need for dietary reforms to reduce their consumption.

Klaunig, J. E., & Kamendulis, L. M. (2004) - The authors explore the role of oxidative stress in cancer development, underscoring the significance of oxidative damage in carcinogenesis.

Aggarwal, B. B., & Gehlot, P. (2009) - This article discusses the relationship between inflammation and cancer, presenting inflammation as a crucial factor in cancer progression and therapy response.

Larsson et al. (2004) - A review that explores potential mechanisms by which dietary long-chain omega-3 fatty acids may prevent cancer, suggesting multiple pathways through which these nutrients exert their effects.

Owen et al. (2000) - This study examines the health benefits of olive oil, particularly its antioxidants, and discusses its potential protective effects against cancer.

DebMandal, M., & Mandal, S. (2011) - The authors provide an overview of the health benefits of coconut, discussing its role in health promotion and disease prevention, including potential anticancer properties.

Fulgoni et al. (2013) - The research highlights the association between avocado consumption and improved diet quality and lower risk of metabolic syndrome, suggesting its role in overall health.

Berries and cancer prevention (2020) - This PubMed article discusses the potential cancer-preventive properties of berries, linking their phytochemical content to reduced cancer risk.

Flavonoids and cancer (2016) - The study reviews the anticancer properties of flavonoids, highlighting their role in cancer prevention and treatment through various biological mechanisms.

Leafy greens and cancer risk (2013) - This article explores the protective effects of leafy greens against cancer, supported by epidemiological evidence linking higher intake to lower cancer risk.

Cruciferous vegetables and cancer (2012) - The research focuses on cruciferous vegetables' potential protective effects against cancer due to their unique compounds, including glucosinolates.

Glucosinolates and cancer (2018) - This study examines glucosinolates found in cruciferous vegetables, discussing their metabolism and potential anticancer effects.

Garlic and cancer prevention (2008) - This article reviews the evidence supporting garlic's role in cancer prevention, emphasizing its bioactive compounds and mechanisms of action.

Organosulfur compounds in garlic (2010) - The research discusses the various organosulfur compounds in garlic and their potential health benefits, including anticancer properties.

Nuts and cancer risk (2018) - This study explores the association between nut consumption and cancer risk, highlighting nuts' role in a healthy diet and potential protective effects.

Seeds and cancer prevention (2017) - The article reviews the health benefits of seeds, including their potential role in cancer prevention, due to their rich nutrient profile.

Green tea and cancer prevention (2008) - This review examines green tea's anticancer properties, focusing on its bioactive compounds and their mechanisms in cancer prevention.

Catechins in green tea (2015) - The study discusses catechins, the primary antioxidants in green tea, and their potential role in cancer prevention.

Lycopene and cancer risk (2013) - This research explores the potential protective effects of lycopene, found in tomatoes, against various types of cancer.

Tomatoes and prostate cancer (2016) - The article discusses the relationship between tomato consumption and reduced prostate cancer risk, emphasizing lycopene's role.

Curcumin and cancer (2019) - This study reviews curcumin's anticancer effects, discussing its mechanisms and potential as a therapeutic agent in cancer treatment.

Turmeric and cancer prevention (2017) - The article examines turmeric's bioactive compounds and their potential role in cancer prevention through various pathways.

Keskin, D., & Kim, Y. J. (2018) - This study investigates the anticancer effects of fenbendazole in a mouse model, providing preliminary insights into its potential as an anticancer agent.

Pantziarka et al. (2014) - The authors discuss the potential of mebendazole as an anti-cancer agent, advocating for its repurposing in oncology.

Clinic for Special Children - This resource provides information about the use of fenbendazole as part of a cancer treatment protocol, outlining its application and context.

Moghadamtousi et al. (2015) - This review explores Annona muricata (graviola), discussing its traditional uses and the biological activities of its isolated acetogenins, including anticancer properties.

Torres et al. (2012) - The study investigates graviola's effects on pancreatic cancer cells, showing its potential to inhibit tumorigenicity and metastasis through metabolic alterations.

Champy et al. (2005) - This research quantifies acetogenins in Annona muricata and discusses their association with atypical parkinsonism, raising concerns about their safety.

National Cancer Institute (NCI) (2021) - This resource provides comprehensive information on antineoplaston therapy, discussing its proposed mechanisms and clinical use.

National Cancer Institute (NCI) (2021) - The NCI outlines laetrile/amygdalin as an alternative cancer treatment, reviewing its history and scientific evaluation.